PRAISE FOR *CIRCLES OF CARE*

◄o►

"Written from within the experience of caregiving, *Circles of Care* recognizes that no one person can handle the strain of caregiving alone, giving many fine suggestions on dealing with the irritation, frustration, and fatigue that inevitably arise. It describes the opportunity that caregivers have to know their subjects intimately and creatively, focusing not on weakness but on strength and on making constructive use of the interests and abilities still available in order to channel the tremendous energy that often remains after nearly everything else is gone."

—MARY MORRISON, author of *Let Evening Come*

"*Circles of Care* is a unique addition to the literature of caregiving, an authoritative and deeply felt book that sheds light on an extraordinary range of eldercare challenges and how to meet them. The book speaks with equal understanding to the experience of the afflicted and those of the family members and caregivers who constitute the 'circle of care.' Being at the center of such a circle or within it, Cason shows us, is part of the privilege of human life."

—AARON ALTERRA, author of *The Caregiver*

CIRCLES
of CARE

HOW TO SET UP
QUALITY HOME CARE
FOR OUR ELDERS

Ann Cason

FOREWORD BY
Reeve Lindbergh

SHAMBHALA
Boston & London
2001

Shambhala Publications, Inc.
Horticultural Hall
300 Massachusetts Avenue
Boston, Massachusetts 02115
www.shambhala.com

9 8 7 6 5 4 3 2 1

First Edition
Printed in the United States of America

∞   This edition is printed on acid-free paper that meets
the American National Standards Institute z39.48 Standard.
Distributed in the United States by Random House, Inc.,
and in Canada by Random House of Canada Ltd.

Library of Congress Cataloging-in-Publication Data
Cason, Ann.
Circles of care : how to set up quality home care for our elders/Ann Cason;
foreword by Reeve Lindbergh.
p.   cm.
Includes bibliographical references and index.
ISBN 1-57062-471-2 (paper: alk. paper)
1. Aged—Home care—United States.   I. Title.
HV1461 .C388   2001
362.6—dc21
00-049655

TO REEVE

who wouldn't let me off the hook

CONTENTS

———◄○►———

FOREWORD

WHEN MY MOTHER, Anne Morrow Lindbergh, first began to show signs of frail old age, I did not think this presented much of a problem. She did the traditionally absentminded things I associated not only with elderly people but also with myself when tired or distracted. She would lose her car keys or her glasses, or perhaps set out to go shopping but find that by the time she reached the store, she had forgotten what she had meant to buy. She might have sudden memory lapses and forget the names of old friends or close family members. ("For heaven's sake! I've known her for fifty years!") I did the same thing myself, sometimes. I still do.

Later, however, her memory trouble was different, and more noticeable. She would call me on the phone in the morning to tell me a funny story, for instance, only it would be exactly the same one she had called to tell me the evening before. She became disoriented in familiar places. Once she completely forgot where she was while standing outside the apartment building of an old friend whom she visited regularly in the city. When the doorman recognized her and spoke to her, she recollected herself, greeted him, and went inside.

My mother has always been courageous. She was quite open about the changes she was noticing in herself as she grew older and was as articulate about the aging process as she had been about every period and experience of her life. She was, at least outwardly, rather amused. She copied out Bette Davis's quotation "Old age is not for sissies" and put it up on her bathroom mirror. She wrote and spoke publicly about aging, at Smith College and at the Cosmopolitan Club in New York City. She called one of her talks "The Tide Flows Out," in what I thought was a wry reference to her best-selling book *Gift from the Sea*. She talked to her family about wanting to write a new book, "a *Gift from the Sea* for old age," and began to research the subject of aging for that purpose. She read works by doctors and by philosophers, by German poets, Buddhist teachers, and Catholic theologians. She wrote a glowing commentary on Florida Scott-Maxwell's candid and passionate memoir about aging, *The Measure of My Days.*

Because she was realistic and practical, my mother had already hired a part-time companion, a young artist friend, to do some driving and some shopping for her on a regular basis. It was understood that this woman would keep track of my mother generally, as needed. It was a warmhearted and unobtrusive arrangement, established in the spirit of friendship, and it was successful for more than a decade.

It was easy, during those years, for my sister and my brothers and me to tell ourselves that our mother was entering old age, yes, but that she would have an easy passage and a quiet journey to an eventual peaceful harbor. That, as I said, was at the very beginning. I was full of assumptions and full of plans. Even at the end of her life, according to these plans, my mother would continue to enrich and illuminate the lives of others, especially mine. As a matter of fact, she has done so, but not quite in the way I had envisioned.

I truly cherished my vision of my mother's old age. I thought it would be a poetic time in both of our lives, a benign and fruitful, slow and mellow season. My mother and I would sit together on the balcony of her home in the sunshine, sipping tea. She would impart wisdom to me with the gentleness of a beloved elder, and I would receive her wisdom with the calm serenity of my mature middle age. I look back on this vision with nostalgic fondness. It was so lovely.

It was also a bunch of baloney, except for the tea. I wasn't wrong about the tea. We do drink a lot of that, and the daily ritual of tea drinking has been a significant part of my mother's life in old age. The rest, however, was sheer fantasy.

What really happened in my mother's frail old age was terrifyingly different from what I had imagined. In her early eighties, my mother's personality seemed to change completely. After suffering a series of strokes, she passed from absentminded forgetfulness into extreme agitation and disorientation, from confusion and anxiety into rage and resistance, and back again. There was not much serenity in my mind, and little apparent in hers, for quite a long time.

When Ann Cason and her circles of care team came into our lives, recommended by a beloved friend of the family who knew Ann and had worked with her in her own family, the atmosphere in my mother's household improved considerably, and her life quieted down a good deal. Over time, with the help of the circle of care Ann established for our mother, we have seen a gradual restoration of a sense of well-being and contentment, even as her health and strength inevitably deteriorate, year by year. Now that she is in her nineties, and very frail indeed, I still have the feeling that my mother has finally come back to herself, returning to a generally peaceful frame of mind.

For my mother and for her whole family, her old age has been an extremely turbulent, active, confusing, and vital time. Without the hard work and generous understanding of Ann Cason and circles of care over the past ten years, I don't know how we would have survived this experience. On the other hand, because we have had Ann's support, along with that of the caregivers she trained, I wouldn't have missed it for anything.

I have learned so much, even though I had to relinquish my dreams and expectations—even though I had to relinquish my mother herself, as I knew her. I have learned that old age and dying definitely are not for sissies, and that they are for us all. I have learned that the ending of a life is not at all what I had thought, and that it does not have to be. I think I may even have learned to be a little less afraid of my own old age, and my own dying, although that remains to be seen.

Ann once told me about a conversation she had with a woman who confessed a lifelong ambition: "to hold the hands of the dying." Ann thought for a while, then laughed and responded, "Well, that's fine, I guess, if you can keep up with them!" This is so true, and so profoundly characteristic of Ann's ability to understand what actually happens, every day, within the real, moment-to-moment experience of someone who is near the end of life, living and dying in his or her own characteristic way: maybe peacefully, maybe not so peacefully; perhaps with passion, perhaps with unrecognized and authentic grace.

Being with a frail old person may not be a matter of sitting quietly by a bedside, holding a hand and smoothing a brow. (It never has been, in my mother's case.) It may be a matter of listening to a flute sonata or listening to a tirade, of taking a drive in the country or hosting a party, of planting flowers, dancing a waltz, or sipping a cup of tea. Sometimes it is all those things in one day, and more, and it always requires as much honest appraisal of oneself as giver of care as it does empathic compassion for the other, the person receiving it.

In this book, Ann Cason shows us not only what a circle of care is and how it operates but also the ways in which a circle of care is presented with many situations, one after another, and how it is possible to work with each one as it comes along. She shows us how the circle of care expands to embrace family members, caregivers, neighbors, friends, and the medical community and how it both challenges and involves each of them. She reveals to us that it is possible to work respectfully with every person whose life is affected by the care situation, and she recognizes that those who give care and those who receive it are not so very different, which may be the most important insight of all.

I know, from my own experience, that the changes that take place when a parent enters frail old age can shake the very foundations of family structure and can cause individual family members to lose their own way in life, at least for a while. This is a tremendously troubling moment for many people, and it casts some of us adrift on uncharted waters, where we must confront mystery and uncertainty and unacknowledged grief and unarticulated fears, all at the same time. Ann Cason's circles of care bring us home again, into a generous, fresh, and gentle approach to caring for our elders, and into a much deeper understanding of ourselves.

REEVE LINDBERGH
May 20, 2000

ACKNOWLEDGMENTS

—◄○►—

M UCH OF WHAT I have learned about working with old people grew
from a partnership with Victoria Howard. We were both living in
Boulder, Colorado, where we had moved to study with Chögyam
Trungpa Rinpoche, founder of Naropa University, who taught us the
basics for working with people. Vicky and I founded and directed a not-
for-profit organization called Dana Home Care, dedicated to helping old
people remain in their own homes. Vicky eventually used her knowledge
about old age to help found the gerontology program at Naropa, to get a
doctorate, and more recently to help found a masters of divinity program
at Naropa to train interfaith chaplains and pastoral caregivers.

One day the Internal Revenue Service came to do an audit of Dana
Home Care. It wanted to see if we were satisfying the requirements to
retain our not-for-profit status. While the auditor sat at a desk poring
over our books, a young care provider came into the office to pick up her
paycheck. "Sharon really enjoyed that ride in the mountains," she told us
cheerfully. "We had such a nice time."

In a flash, the auditor sprang from her desk and came over to where
Vicky and I were sitting. "Are you wasting the taxpayers' money taking
old people for rides?" she asked sternly. "Oh, no," Vicky told her, as I fid-
dled with my pencil. "We'd never take an old person for a ride. We were
just returning from a doctor's appointment."

"Well, that's OK," the auditor said, and walked back to her desk.

As she sat down, I thought to myself, "It's all upside down." And it's
worse today. We're afraid to spend a penny on well-being, but we throw
away billions of dollars on mood elevators and CT scans and operations,
in an attempt to mop up the misery of fragile lives. In the end, there is little money for good care, the kind that helps the spirits soar. But Vicky

knew what the auditor didn't: old people and their helpers have to learn to be in simple ways—an ice cream on the way back from the doctor, a quiet drive in the countryside, breathing in the freshness of an autumn day, or just sitting silently and watching the sun glisten on the back of a blackbird's wing. These beliefs inspired me to write this book, and Vicky exemplified them.

Many other people have participated in the writing of this book: the elders who have shared their lives by letting themselves be cared for, the many caregivers who have shared their wisdom about taking care, and those who have given me support along the way with their writing, organizational, and editorial skills.

Old age itself is fairly simple, but what goes on around it is complex. It takes a great deal of energy, discipline, and joy on the part of caregivers to keep from sinking into a state of mind that yields to despair and feels burdened. I asked myself, "After taking care of old people for ten years, how hard could it be to write a book?" However, I found that giving birth to a book is not easy. Many people helped me along the way. Robert Hirshfield showed me how to write sentences. At one point when I had hundreds of pages of manuscript, Toinette Lippe and Katharine LeMee gave me assistance and encouragement. Helen Berliner was very helpful. When I had given up and stuffed the whole thing into a big, black garbage bag, Jim and Ellen Green encouraged me. When it was sorted out, Jane Fuller read it and made suggestions. Beth Dugger read it and loved it and invited me into the writing group to which she belonged, which was Reeve Lindbergh's End of the Road writing group. All of its members have provided so much support, both by intelligent reading and by expressing the attitude "You can do it." So I am especially grateful to Liz Truslow, Sheila Reed, Melinda Evans, Amy Ehrlich, Catherine Soares, and Carol Hyman. Also, thanks to Peggy Jennings for her reading of the manuscript and her intelligent comments. My appreciation to Vicky Giella for the clarification of many fine points. And finally, when the "baby" was far enough along, my gratitude to Emily Hilburn Sell, the senior editor at Shambhala Publications, and to Joel Segel and Holly Hammond.

Thanks to the many caregivers with whom I have connected over the past twentysome years. There are too many to list, but I would like to especially express my appreciation to the early helpers at Dana Home Care: Ellie Kraemer, R.N.; Mary Schumacher; Katherine Campbell; Sondra Field; Maggie Donaghy; Reva Tift; Nancy Castleberry; Bill and Diane Brauer; Susan Kessler; and although she has not lived to see this thanks, Kay Landt. I see all of you in these pages.

In more recent years, I have learned so much from Susan Drommond, Laurie Crosby, Alexandra Evans, Buncie Shadden, Carla Leftwich, Sue Gilman, Catherine Clark, Susan Shaw, Karen Frasier, Phil Sentner, John Hopkins, and the very fine hospice nurse Arthur Jennings. Many thanks to the doctors who shared their wisdom about caring for the old from the medical perspective: Ed Podvall, Mitchell Levy, Phil Weber, Greg Rabold, and Tim Thompson (to name only a few).

I'm indebted, as well, to Margot Wilkie, who opened my world in many directions, and to Anne Morrow Lindbergh, who in her great wisdom and ability to communicate has demonstrated the spirit of old age.

I would also like to thank my family: my mother, Mary Lois Adams, who was spared from old age by dying quickly at the age of sixty-five; my father, Clifford Adams, who was so thrilled about this book; and his dear wife, Eleanor, who took such kind and thoughtful care of him for so many years. I also want to express my gratitude to my two sisters, Jane Jenkins and Judy Craig. Somehow we made it through our father's old age loving one another. And most of all, I want to thank Fred Cason, who supported me in so many ways during the making of *Circles of Care,* as well as my son, Eric Cason, who can barely remember a time in his life when I wasn't working on "the book." I hope he will find it helpful when it is his turn to care for me.

INTRODUCTION

———◄o►———

I ONCE VISITED AN OLD COUPLE who lived in a high-rise apartment on the shore of a large lake. The husband had suffered a series of small strokes, which left him slow-moving and slightly befuddled. When I arrived, he sat at the dining room table surrounded by his wife, his daughter, his son, and a caregiver. The atmosphere in the room was heavy with unspoken conflict.

The wife had bought her husband some new clothes, as if to ensure that he would not die and leave her. The daughter didn't like the new clothes; she wanted her father to dress as he had always dressed, so he would always be her same old father. The son was remembering, with distress, the voice of the doctor saying, "We won't use heroic measures to keep him alive." The caregiver was concerned about following the advice of the visiting nurse, who wanted to change the man's diet, and of the physical therapist, who wanted him to do more exercise. Then the old man said to his wife, "Why do we need all this help when you have me to take care of you?"

I sat there wondering how I could help. Could I find a way to meet the elder's care needs while relaxing the family's struggle? How could I begin to tackle this complex tangle of emotional and practical problems? Then the family showed me their way.

The teakettle began to whistle from the kitchen, and the sadness was dispelled. The daughter poured hot water into a white china teapot and brought out a platter of pastries and bright napkins. As we ate, the sun struck the lake and reflected through the window. That moment of relaxation was the first step toward creating a circle of care. We did not have to solve problems or put a lid on conflict. As everyone relaxed, a workable plan came into being.

The ebbing of the life force is a genuine and precious part of human experience, but we are not usually prepared for it. To those of us who are witnessing someone's decline, it is like standing on the beach at night, watching the tide roll out: lonely, haunting, and hard to fathom. This powerful atmosphere often reveals what has been hidden in someone's life. It bares the heart and mind and soul. It shows the many faces of love and how a person has expressed it or run from it. It shows the blows of fate that life has dealt and all the ways that a person has yielded or taken a stand. These revelations are the starting point of care.

Being old is a major life shift. The elder is required to go from doing into being. Many of us have lived life going full steam ahead, always engaged in activity. Old age requires a change in that pace. It may come on gradually, as energy and memory decline, or it may come abruptly, with illness or the loss of a mate. The atmosphere turns gray and heavy; the ground is littered with shards of broken dreams.

On the day I found out that this book had been accepted for publication, I ran into a friend at a meeting. As I told him about the book, he stopped me in midsentence. "Well, it should have a good market," he said. Then his face turned red and he clenched his fists. "It is so irritating."

As my friend then shared with me his strong feelings about taking care of his mother, I wanted to wrap him in the embrace of all the wonderful sons, daughters, spouses, health care professionals, ministers, friends, and neighbors who have been part of a circle of care for someone old. Those of us who have learned directly from elderly people want to share our experiences with those of you who are starting on the path of care. This book is primarily addressed to families of elders who need care. It will also give experienced caregivers a fresh approach to their work.

Circles of Care will take you through exercises, care studies, and suggestions to help you understand how old age feels and how you can help. Your sadness and irritation are understandable. If you have tried to protect yourself from strong feelings as your loved one has grown frail, you may have become numb. Irritation is a sign that the numbness is leaving, like a sleeping foot beginning to tingle as circulation is restored. Irritation is enlivening; it wakes you, shakes you, and fills you with energy.

With this energy, you will be able to take care of your parent, spouse, or client. You will learn to see yourself as more than arms and legs and eyes of the person for whom you're caring, as more than a custodian of the helpless. You will become a protector of the elder's being. You will learn to accept what is and to make it as good as you can. You will begin to see old people not only as provokers of anxiety but also as teachers who are taking their caregivers on a journey of the heart. In the process, you will be touched by the goodness of life, a life that includes the knowing of death.

BEFORE YOU START

B EFORE YOU START THINKING about the details of caretaking, close your eyes and picture yourself sitting with your aging parent or spouse. Other family members are there. You are sitting in folding chairs in a small room with tile floors, beige walls, and bright fluorescent lights. Imagine that you are all arguing with one another. Each person has a different opinion. Make the arguments as realistic as you can.

For example, one person might say, "Well, she made her bed, let her lie in it." Another says that pneumonia is the old person's friend; don't give her medicine. One person says that she has to care for her mother in the way that her mother cared for her. Another says no, you have to take care of yourself. Someone else says that she has no time or money. The elder says that she doesn't want help. A son says it is hopeless. A daughter says that death is natural, and we should let it be. One person says that we have to fight this with all available technology. Another says that the symptoms of old age are the sign of an imbalance, and he wants to use body work and homeopathic remedies. A brother says that it is time for his sister to let go and die.

Let yourself feel pulled in more than one direction. Let yourself feel angry, closed in, tense, bewildered, perched on the hard chairs with the fluorescent lights glaring down.

Then imagine that the room and the chairs and the lights all fall away. Instead of sitting in a room, you are in a meadow. You still have the same concerns, but you are sitting on green grass surrounded by wildflowers. Hills can be seen off in the distance. Birds are flying and singing. The sky is clear and blue, with an occasional cloud floating by. How do you feel now?

Sit in the meadow and ask yourself these questions: Is it possible to find well-being in the midst of illness? Do I see confusion or poor health as signs of failure? Do I think that the elder ended up old and sick because he did something wrong? Could what we call dementia simply be a different way of looking at the world?

Do I find myself trying to fix things that cannot be fixed? Do I want to shield myself and my loved one from mortality? Should death be kept private? Should a person be willing to share her dying with others?

Can I see working with frailty as a way to learn more about myself? Am I afraid to ask for help? Do I see love as sacrifice or as a way to move beyond solitary strength and open out to others?

PART ONE

—◄○►—

THE BASICS

CHAPTER 1

———◄○►———

Entering the Elder's World

M Y FATHER WAS AN ENTREPRENEUR who pioneered new products and developed many businesses. Work had been his life. His pleasure was getting up early and writing out his plans and dreams on yellow pads. When he lost his health, he had to give up his business. His memory failed, and he lost his ability to be a provider. He had always been cheerful and optimistic when facing big obstacles in life, but this time he sank and couldn't recover. He began to spend his days sitting in an easy chair watching television. Since he could no longer drive, his second wife, Eleanor, fifteen years younger and still working, had to leave her job every time he needed to go to the doctor or wanted to go swimming. The only stimulation my father could find in his narrowing world was trying to win millions of dollars from *Reader's Digest* or Publisher's Clearing House.

After spending a week with my father, I wrote down his daily schedule. Here is what it looked like:

5:00 to 6:00 AM	Gets up and makes own breakfast, brings in paper.
6:00 to 7:00	Showers and shaves.
7:00 to 8:00	Watches "Today Show" on TV.
8:00 to 11:00	Watches CNN, reads headlines, dozes.
11:00 to 11:30	Drinks diet Coke.
11:30 to 12:30 PM	Works on papers from *Reader's Digest* contest.
12:30 to 1:00	Makes lunch, sets table, waits for wife to come home from work.

1:00 to 2:00	Eats lunch, talks to wife, who is home for lunch.
2:00 to 3:00	Dozes in front of television.
3:00 to 5:00	Has a doctor's appointment, goes swimming, or waits for wife to come home.
6:00 to 7:00	Eats supper.
7:00 to 9:00	Watches television and dozes until bedtime.

As I considered my father's daily life, it appeared that he had lost his footing as a productive member of society. He couldn't accept this loss, so he began to live in a dream world. But perhaps I wasn't looking closely enough. It's important not to make quick judgments about another person's life. The task is to see where a person is connected to and disconnected from his basic sense of himself.

To look more deeply at who the elder is, ask what he or she truly cares about. Is it family, work, raising children? Did she want to travel? Did he want to find true love? Has she been driven by the desire to make the world a better place? Has he been on a lifelong search for truth and beauty or the meaning of life? Did she need to express herself artistically? What was his mission in life? What was her idea of success? Maybe he just wanted to do what was right under his nose and look no farther.

LOOKING THREE WAYS

To discover a person's reason for living and basic motivation, it helps to look at three aspects of life: physical expression, relationships, and state of mind.

First, look at the physical side of life. Is the person's house or room well tended or cluttered? Is it safe? Does it let in light? Does it accommodate visitors, or does it try to keep them away? Is the house full of magazines or books? Are the walls covered with works of art or pictures of family? How is the person dressed? What are his ailments, his daily routines? What does she hear, see, taste, smell, and touch? What are her food preferences? What routines make the elder feel safe or isolated?

Next, look at the elder's relationships. Does he have relationships with family, tradespeople, pets? What about friends and doctors? Who makes the elder feel nurtured or abandoned? Is she alone most of the time? How does he relate to his world? Is he angry? Is he collapsed in bed with the covers over his head? Is she manipulative? Does she long for the past?

Then consider the elder's state of mind. Is it settled or chaotic? Is she relaxed or agitated, spaced-out or present, clear or confused? What makes him feel upset or calm, crazy or sane?

If you don't know what an elder is thinking or feeling, pay attention to the atmosphere that surrounds her. Especially notice how you feel when you are with her. Someone may be smiling and telling you that everything is fine, but you notice that you feel nervous or oppressed. You may be experiencing the feelings that the elder is trying to hide. Of course, that same process may work in reverse: if you are trying to hide your feelings, the elder might experience them.

It isn't easy to get an overview of another's life. When you look at a person's situation, you might tend to latch onto one detail, name it as the problem, and try to find a solution. For instance, if someone has diabetes, it is a relief to know what to do: diet, foot care, medicine. This could be the starting point of care, but you shouldn't stop there. Look at the elder and his world from different angles, without trying to resolve anything yet. The care plan will evolve, starting from the elder's needs.

As I looked at my father's life in these three ways, I saw the pride he took in having learned to make his own breakfast and lunch. When my mother died, he hadn't known how to boil an egg. His lunch now was meager, but it seemed to satisfy him. His routines had become all-important to him, not just as a substitute for companionship but also as his discipline.

Relationship was focused on his second wife, Eleanor. This heart connection was very important, but I wondered if he needed contact with more people. He had a few visitors from the church, but his family lived far away, and many of his friends had died. Next to Eleanor, his doctors became his most constant friends.

It was in my father's state of mind that the difficulty lay. He would tell me that he felt fine and would live forever, but the atmosphere around him was pervaded by a sense of doom. He would pace the floor waiting for the mail carrier to come. Then he'd sort through the mail looking for papers from a contest. He was obsessed with contests, and his delusion was leading him toward isolation.

As I looked at the way my father lived his life, I was filled with tenderness and fear and the heart-wrenching desire to fix it. At the same time, I respected the way that he was managing. He had been such a doer, always making things happen, and now he was up against something very basic. He—and I—had to learn to be with his life as it was.

It is easy to think that we know what another person should do. But the task for the caregiver is to see and accept what the elder is showing you. With my own father, it took me a long time to understand his motivations.

LOOKING TO THE ELDER'S STRENGTHS

When someone needs your care, it is easy to focus on the difficulties he or she is facing and not pay enough attention to the person's abilities. My father's strengths were his disciplined schedule, a good relationship with his wife, and his love of swimming. Swimming made him feel strong and energized, and talking to people at the swim club connected him to a larger world. After swimming, he would buy a diet Coke and sit and relax. He felt a part of the vigor swirling around him at the club. For the rest of the day, he would forget that he needed to win a million dollars.

I wanted to support what made my father feel most connected to life. In consultation with my sisters, we worked out a plan to hire a driver (from a home-care agency) to take my father swimming. The driver would also take him to the doctor, so that Eleanor would not have to leave work to do it. Our hope was that removing a burden from his wife and encouraging his activity might also have the effect of promoting his sense of well-being and thereby lessen his obsession with contests.

You are one of the elder's strengths as well; otherwise, you would not be reading this book. Listen to yourself and your siblings or anyone else who will be involved in the elder's care. Hear their concerns. You may not agree on what course to take. You may worry that your parent doesn't have the money for care. You may feel humiliated that you have not escaped from your parent's net. You may feel helpless if your parent lives far away or if you can't resolve his delusions. You may have to face living with a sense of impending disaster.

If you try to establish a plan of care prematurely and then struggle to carry it out, you will end up fighting a losing battle with the elder or with your siblings. Then, instead of a circle of care, you end up with an arena in which the lions are chasing the gladiators. You can save yourself time and heartache in the long run if you spend some time looking, listening, and contemplating as the first stage of care. Maybe you won't be able to change very much, but you will see the issues more clearly, and the clarity itself will lead the way to a plan.

THE CIRCLE OF CARE

Have you ever walked outside on a spring day to see the first crocuses poking their green shoots up from the ground? Remember when you were sick and your mother brought you a bowl of soup? For a moment, your spirits lifted, and your problems dissolved. You felt webs of connection invisible to the naked eye. These are the connections that will weave a circle of care around you and the old person in your care. They will take the form of a trustworthy inner voice or an auspicious coincidence: just the right helper will arrive, a book will fall into your hand, a friend will tell you about an agency that helped her mother.

We want to see the elder surrounded by a circle of care: family and helpers, friends and neighbors, and all the professional people—the doctor, the nurse, the lawyer, the social worker, the minister or rabbi. The circle will include others as well: the mail carrier, the grocer, the hairdresser or barber. A circle of care embraces whatever feelings or events come along: anger, joy, sadness, illness, and grief. The goal is not to change anyone but to let all of our various agendas relax into awareness and acceptance. The circle helps both elder and caregivers feel at home, wherever that may be.

EXERCISE: *Telling the Elder's Story*

———◄○►———

Here is an exercise to help expand your usual way of thinking about your loved one. Ask a friend who does not know the elder to witness your presentation of him or her. Start with a physical description of the person, the house, and the neighborhood. Pretend that you are writing a novel or a play and want to bring this character to life. Forget who you are and let yourself slip inside the old person's skin. Walk to the bathroom on her legs; lie down on her bed. If the person is bent, bend over and look out at the world from that angle. If she is blind, cover your eyes and feel around. Tell her life story from her point of view: "I grew up in Kansas and met my husband when I was eighteen. When he died, I didn't know who I was." Tell what your journey in life has been, with its strengths and obstacles. Let yourself feel her emotions and state of mind.

After your presentation, let your friend ask you questions, and answer them as best you can. See if you don't have a better sense of the elder and her world. What are her strengths? What obstacles does she face? Don't try to resolve the obstacles. Later, when the circle of care develops, you will meet those obstacles again. Maybe your understanding will help them to relax.

CARE STUDY

Listening and Letting Go

————◀◦▶————

Pearl lived alone in a little white house. After a life in Iowa, where she and her husband had farmed and operated a small café, the widowed Pearl moved to Colorado to be near her grown children. But at age eighty-eight, Pearl's increasing isolation and frailty led her to a life of complaint. Day after day, she sat in her rocking chair lamenting, "What is this world coming to?" She complained about her painful knees, about her failing eyesight, and about Lucille and Jack, her grown children.

The neighbors were concerned, and Jack and Lucille wondered what to do. Jack worried about Pearl's safety and thought she should live in a nursing home. Lucille worried about finances and wanted Pearl to stay in her own home until she died. Pearl's doctor had told them that their mother's heart and lungs were ruined and that she needed constant care.

When Lucille visited her mother, the curtains and windows were closed in the stuffy room. The lace-covered table beside her mother's chair was piled with pill bottles, stacks of papers, and a little crystal tree. Pearl told her daughter once again about running the café in Iowa. Lucille imagined her mother as she had been in the past, and she was overcome with sadness. She wanted to leave.

As Lucille prepared to go, her mother switched on the crystal tree. Lucille looked at the twinkling lights, then met Pearl's eyes. In a flash, her depression faded, and she felt a deep connection to her mother. Lucille sat back down. Pearl reminisced about their pond in Iowa, where giant birds swooped down at dusk.

Later, in my office, Lucille told Jack, "You know, on my last visit to mother, something happened to me. At first, I felt so depressed, I thought I would die. Then I stayed for an hour, and something clicked. I had a great time." As Jack and Lucille talked, I remembered another old woman and her family.

Sharon, who belittled her daughter and fought with her son, had been a difficult person all her life. With old age, she became more so. Her son brought Sharon to Colorado to live near him in a rented apartment. She had helpers around the clock, and he visited her frequently. But family conflict intensified.

Sharon whined and moaned, and her son shouted, "Mother, you don't have to be so neurotic." While he paced the floor of her living room, Sharon threatened, "I'm going to kill myself." She was insatiable in the demands she made upon her family and helpers.

While Sharon raged and complained, the helpers cooked and cleaned. When Sharon repeated herself, the helpers took turns listening to her. In the gaps between her various complaints, caregivers took Sharon for drives in the country, took her out to dinner, and helped her with her passion in life—writing poetry. They also gave parties for Sharon and her family.

So it went for a couple of years. One evening Sharon said to her son, "You never do what I ask." It was at a party for the son, his wife, and a few friends and caregivers. Wine flowed, and the radio blared a country tune about going out in a blaze of glory and all good things coming to an end. "I want you to dance," Sharon said.

Jack looked at her, all his old exasperation rising again in his face. Then something cleared, and he got to his feet and began a slow, rhythmic dance around the room. As the beat picked up, he whirled faster. He danced for his mother and for all the old people in the world who need care. Then he sat back down. The frenzied irritation between mother and son relaxed into the sadness and grace of the dance.

A few days later, Sharon fell into a coma. It seemed as if the son's yielding to the spirit of the moment had allowed his mother to go forward. He hadn't just obeyed a request; he had participated in a celebration. For years this mother and son had been locked in struggle. The son, by yielding to what the situation required of him, had helped them both past the deadlock. Although parents sometimes demand the impossible from their children, circles of care can create the support that helps people relax and move forward.

My attention came back to the present moment, in which Jack and Lucille were deciding to keep Pearl in her own home and to bring in helpers. But a few weeks later, they sat in my office once more. "I wish I could control my mother," Lucille said as she paced the floor. "Now, Lucille," consoled Jack, "you got that nice girl to live in part-time, you got the visiting nurse, you got the home-care agency to fix her meals and clean. You're doing what you can."

"But Mom wants the live-in to use her dirty bathwater. She won't let the girl use butter on her toast, and now she's saying she doesn't need help. She'd rather go die in a hospital."

While Lucille and Jack talked, I thought about how the genuine connection between parents and grown children so often leads to conflict. Pearl and Lucille hadn't learned to appreciate their boundaries, their differences. Pearl had been a helper to her husband, a mother to her children. She had stayed in the same place most of her life. But Lucille was different—a traveler and a scholar. The differences between them, instead of igniting communication, had bogged them down. "You should be a wife and mother," Pearl would say. To her, this was a compliment. She loved Lucille and wanted the same life for her as she, Pearl, had had. Lucille stayed away from Pearl so she wouldn't criticize her mother's narrow opinions or lose her temper. This was her way of helping. When mother and daughter did get together, each tried to control the other with her fantasies of what she thought the other should become. They didn't realize that they were two separate people, each with her own journey in life.

People often define themselves through the feedback they get from others. When the accustomed feedback is not forthcoming, there is loneliness and a feeling of abandonment. A writer or a teacher may define himself through the eyes of the public. When that audience is no longer there, he might fill the empty space with excessive routines and old habits. A social person or a family person might see herself through the eyes of her friends or children. If she is too weak to give a party, or if the family is scattered, she feels abandoned and may complain excessively. A wife may define her existence through the eyes of her husband. If her husband dies, she may grieve not only for him but for her own role in life.

If you haven't discovered how the elder defines herself or himself, you may stumble as you attempt to communicate. Pearl had always been a helper, and she still wanted to help. But she was old and sick and couldn't even take care of herself anymore. The more she became disconnected from her accustomed way of being, the more Pearl tried to control others. Unable to see herself as worthwhile, Pearl retreated into her self-absorbed thoughts, which became her reality. "Jack is a good boy. Lucille is a bad girl. Richard Nixon let us down. I just can't see." Pearl's world had narrowed to those few sentences.

Fortunately, all self-images can shift. A circle of care can start with a closed-in world of isolation, then expand to intersect with other worlds. Many frail people have a few sentences and a few routines that seem to be the sum total of their existence, but that world is not solid. One minute Pearl is complaining about her daughter, the next she wants a cherry Coke, the next she relaxes into the accommodating silence.

It is important to listen to the details of the elder's world, to enter that world fully for a moment, but not to take it too seriously. As Lucille and Jack spent more time with their mother and listened to her worries, they saw that Pearl's figments hid something tender and worth knowing. Looking back on her life, listening to her concerns, noticing the framed certificates of gratitude from organizations she'd helped over the years, they understood that caring had always been Pearl's concern. She'd been a helper all her life; now she was having trouble accepting help. Jack and Lucille became more gentle with Pearl in discussing her concerns. Could the woman who lived in be allowed to have her own bathwater? Might she have butter on her toast?

One winter afternoon, the phone rang in my office. "Pearl is dying," the caregiver told me over the phone. I drove over to Pearl's house. She lay on her antique bed with her eyes closed. While I sat with Pearl, Jack went into the next room to phone Lucille, who was off in another town. "Pearl is very ill," Jack whispered into the phone. "Please come. We need you." Pearl looked up at me and asked, "Is she coming?" Before I could answer, Pearl struggled to get up and sat in the rocking chair, where she rocked and waited.

I went back to my office and reported to the doctor. "Congestive heart failure," he said. "She would be more comfortable in the hospital. Her lungs are filling up."

Back at Pearl's, Jack and I sat with her. Cautiously, Jack broached the subject. "Pearl, the doctor says your heart is worn out." "Well, I can't help it. My knees hurt. I can't see," Pearl said. "Mother, the doctor says it doesn't look too good," Jack explained. "He thinks he can make you more comfortable in the hospital, but Lucille says you'd be better off at home."

Pearl rocked a little faster. A tissue fell out of the pocket of her house-coat. I reached down to pick it up. Jack said, "We don't know what you want, Mother. Do you want to go to the hospital or stay home?" "Well, if the doctor says I should go to the hospital, I guess I should," Pearl replied.

Pearl went to the hospital, and in a few days the doctor called to say that she could come home. Lucille brought her home and put her to bed. "Ma, I want you to stay home," Lucille told her. Pearl turned her head to the wall. "Mother, it's not just the money. I want to be here with you." Jack took Pearl's hand.

Jack and Lucille had learned to let go of their opinions and give what was genuinely required. They created a circle of care, a healing environ-ment, which helped them gain insight as they came to understand Pearl's needs and their own. First, they met the practical requirements of the sit-uation, then in the midst of resistance, irritation, and love, they went for-ward. They overcame their need to change their mother. They went through their fear of her depression and complaints to open ground, where anything could happen.

As I walked out the door, it was snowing heavily, and my car was stuck. Walking home, I said to myself, "Here I am in Colorado, where it snows all the time, and we don't even have enough snowplows in this town." Then I caught myself sounding just like Pearl. So I simply walked, listening to the sound of snow crunching under my boots.

CHAPTER 2

———◄○►———

Getting Help

WHEN YOUR LOVED ONE NEEDS CARE, you need people to help you. You don't know how long their help will be required or how the elder's situation might change over time. Every old person's life is different. Some people can get by with only a little support at certain times of the day. But if that limited help is not provided, they may become so anxious or confused that much more attention becomes necessary. So you must develop a circle of care that will be reliable, with backup contingencies to deal with the unexpected, and flexible, to meet changing needs—a circle that will perform compassion's work and will support both the elder and you.

Creating a circle of care is like working on a puzzle. It takes diligence as well as bursts of inspiration. Keeping the atmosphere of an old person's world light, warm, friendly, and accommodating is best accomplished through a coordinated effort of family, caretakers, and agencies. You may want to hire a professional care coordinator if you can afford it. But even with a manager, it is good for the family to have a sense of the rhythm of the elder's life, because professional helpers are only one part of the circle of care.

ASSESSING THE ELDER'S EVERYDAY NEEDS

Start by writing down the elder's daily schedule, noting what happens during each hour of the day. Notice the level of energy, the habits and routines, the existing interests, and what resources are already in place. In my experience, it is the best map to help a caregiver look at an elder's life. Later it will become a tool of communication with the old person.

If you are a spouse, maybe you already know the schedule so well that it is difficult to stand back and actually see it. If you are a caregiver starting with a new client, it sometimes takes a while to recognize the rhythm of the daily schedule. But it's a good place to start, because it lets you see what you have to work with.

Once you've identified the basic components of the schedule, indicate the points at which you think help is (or is not) needed, as in the following example:

6:00 to 7:00 AM	Gets up.	Can manage alone.
7:00 to 8:00	Eats breakfast.	Can manage alone.
8:00 to 10:00	Performs personal care.	Needs help.
10:00 to 12:00 N	Rests.	Can manage alone.
12:00 to 1:00 PM	Eats lunch.	Needs help.
1:00 to 4:00	Rests.	Can manage alone.
4:00 to 5:00	Sorts papers.	Can manage alone.
5:00 to 6:00	Has tea.	Friends often come.
6:00 to 7:00	Eats dinner.	Needs help.
7:00 to 9:00	Reads, watches TV.	Can manage alone.
9:00 to 10:00	Prepares for bed.	Can manage alone.
10:00 to 2:00 AM	Sleeps.	Can manage alone.
2:00 to 2:30	Goes to bathroom.	Can manage alone.
2:30 to 6:00	Sleeps lightly.	Can manage alone.

When you look at this schedule, you can see that the person requires help with personal care and meals. There may be other needs as well, but start with the most obvious. Sometimes when the basic needs are met, other issues sort themselves out. With this schedule, you might want a caregiver to come each day from 9:00 AM to 1:00 PM. The duties would be to help with bathing and dressing, perform light household chores, fix and serve lunch, and prepare a meal to leave for dinner. The helper would also

schedule beauty and doctor's appointments, provide transportation, and
do the weekly shopping and meal planning.

Now step back and consider other things that need to be done less frequently—weekly, biweekly, monthly. Pay close attention to the involve-
ment of friends, neighbors, relatives, and other caregivers in the elder's
life. Does someone come to mow the lawn? Is there a bookkeeper? Who
cleans the house? Who does the shopping? All of these helpers should be
taken into account when assessing the basic circle of care.

DETERMINING THE RANGE OF AVAILABLE SERVICES

You can hire a helper or put together a combination of helpers and community services. Two sources for information on services in the community are the Area Agency on Aging and the senior center. They will be
able to connect you with whoever is in charge of information and assistance. The information-and-assistance position was funded by the Older
Americans Act in 1965, so most Area Agencies on Aging have such a position. If your local Area Agency on Aging doesn't, you can reach an Eldercare Locator toll-free at (800) 677-1116.

The following services are available in many communities free of
charge:

- *Telephone reassurance*: A volunteer calls the elderly person each
  morning and reports back to the agency that provides the service if
  there is no answer.
- *Senior companion*: Trained senior companions visit the elderly.
- *Senior transportation*: Drivers take elders to medical appointments
  or other supportive services.

The following fee-based services are often available as well:

- *Hot meals*: Nourishing meals are delivered to homebound old people
  five times a week. On Friday two extra meals may be left for the
  weekend. The charge for this service, which is sometimes called
  Meals on Wheels, is on a sliding scale, based on the elder's income.

- *Congregate meals*: Some organizations serve group meals to the elderly for a reasonable price.
- *Day care*: Some organizations provide daytime care and offer other activities for the elderly. The charge for day care is usually reasonable, with the fee sometimes being on a sliding scale, based on income.
- *Licensed home health care*: Nursing, physical therapy, home health aides, homemakers, and other Medicare-covered services are provided.
- *Private homemaker agency*: Homemakers and personal-care attendants are provided.
- *Assisted-living or residential homes*: Usually, meals, personal care, and activities are provided.
- *Nursing home*: Complete care, including skilled nursing, is provided.
- *Senior center*: Social and cultural activities are held, and information and referrals can be obtained.
- *Support groups*: Such groups are available for caregivers as well as for people with Alzheimer's, diabetes, Parkinson's disease, and other disorders.
- *Care coordination or management*: A trained individual sets up and manages care programs within an elder's home. The coordinator or manager helps families make decisions about the elder's needs and assists with details of carrying out the plan. To find a care manager, ask the local Area Agency on Aging, which will know about private care managers or may be able to provide case management services if the elder is eligible for Medicaid. (The Area Agency on Aging can provide counseling and do assessments of the elder's needs and finances to determine what assistance he or she is eligible for.) The National Association of Professional Geriatric Care Managers also provides a directory, available by calling (520) 881-8008 or through its Web site, at www.caremanager.org. Small local agencies also provide care coordination. Finally, you might try advertising in the paper for a person who would like to try care coordinating using this book as a guide.

You might be tempted to line up only one helper or try to manage by yourself. But the advantages of creating a small caregiving team far outweigh the disadvantages. One caregiver can easily lose her sense of humor, while two or three people keep things lively. It's easy to become overly dependent on a single helper, and there is great risk of overburdening everyone involved. The team approach is especially useful when problems arise, and it helps prevent burnout. A group brings balance and accountability as well as a variety of skills and points of view. Providing twenty-four-hour care may take anywhere from three to six people a week.

The Care Coordinator or Manager

Helpers and services can come together in many different ways to form the basic circle of care. The one who pulls it all together is the coordinator or manager. This might be a paid coordinator, an agency, or a family member. Sometimes different family members take turns coordinating. The person who coordinates hires and works with staff, decides on the plan of care, and sees that the details of the plan are carried out. The coordinator arranges for trips to the hairdresser or doctor, finds a replacement when one helper is sick, explains the routines to helpers, and makes decisions about purchases and changing needs.

The coordinator also helps to settle the conflicts that will inevitably arise. An old man wants cream on his cereal, but the caregivers want to give him skim milk. One caregiver wants to get an elder up at 8:00 AM; the other wants to let her sleep. One helper wants to buy a blender; the other wants a bouquet of flowers; another says, "Forget flowers; the old person needs a psychiatrist." These issues, which might seem small, are at the heart of home care. If there is no format for discussion and resolution, members of the team will battle it out. The coordinator is there to do whatever is necessary to resolve such issues so that injured feelings don't harden into resentment.

The manager needs to be a strong person who is willing to say yes or no. But sometimes a solution comes out of a team meeting, at which issues are discussed until a consensus is reached. One old woman had diabetes, and there was a disagreement within her care team about her diet. The woman wanted chocolate cake. Her son said, "Let her have the cake. Isn't is better to die at feast than at famine?" The visiting nurse said that the elder might end up blind or with amputated limbs. In the team meeting, a plan was worked out: the caregivers would cook the diabetic diet, which would include a very small piece of cake. Everybody on the team had to empathize with the woman's longing, talk to her about her diet, and turn their heads if she sneaked a bite of cake at a party.

Care coordinators need to be intimately involved with the issues that come up in an old person's world. An ideal way to do this is for the coordinator to provide some of the care, or to start the care and then add other helpers as they are needed, although often coordinators don't have the time to work shifts. (I discuss more about how to supervise circles of care in Chapter 4.)

Many nurses and social workers, as well as some gerontologists and psychologists, offer care-coordination services. They charge from $30 per hour to $100 per hour in major cities. But a person who is interested, organized, and good at working with people can learn to be a care coordinator.

Hiring Helpers

If you're working as the care coordinator, you are responsible for finding good helpers. Some care coordinators use agencies to find helpers. If you don't want to use an agency, look for likely candidates in your immediate surroundings. Someone you already know—a neighbor or an acquaintance—might want some work. The elder might have a friend who needs a little extra cash. Perhaps the man who mows the lawn knows a woman who is looking for work. Tell everyone you know that you are looking for someone to join your circle of care. Put up notices on the bulletin boards of churches, grocery stores, self-service laundries, meditation centers, and colleges. Give a clear description of the job and include your phone number. If you advertise in the newspaper, indicate what the job consists of and what type of person you are seeking. Be sure to stress that you are looking for a team member. A team approach tends to discourage undesirables who prey upon the elderly.

Home-care workers are required to have a certain number of hours of training before they can work in nursing homes or Medicare-certified home-care agencies. But sometimes people without training make just as effective helpers. Domestic and personal-care skills are easy to learn. Those who see taking care of old people not as a profession but as a way to earn money while doing something useful are sometimes easier to work with.

When people begin to call in response to your search, have a long phone conversation with each one. Discourage people with whom you don't connect. Invite people you like to come for an interview.

Trust your feelings. Don't hire anyone unless you would enjoy being with that person yourself. Include the elder in the hiring process as much as possible. Old people are often shrewd judges of character. In any case, the chemistry has to be right in a caregiving relationship. If the elder is not included in the process of hiring, he might feel that his independence is being stolen and try to subvert the care. I found this out in my early days of caretaking.

I was calling on ministers of churches, telling them about our home-care service, when one minister said to me, "Well, that sounds good, but I hear that you ladies have been stealing from Alice Jackson." I went to Alice's house to talk to her about the complaint. "What has been stolen from you, Alice?" I asked. "Well," she said, "there was half a sweet roll in the back of my refrigerator that is missing, and there were two paper clips in that bowl on my desk. And those girls you sent make me get down on my knees to pray every day." Alice hadn't been included in the decision about her care, and she tried everything in her power to get rid of her helpers. This doesn't mean that you can't insist on care for frail elders, but you have to be prepared for the consequences.

When you find someone you want to hire, make sure that the job description is as clear as you can make it and that the length of commitment is understood. Plan to pay a reasonable wage, and institute a system so that helpers receive their pay on time. Think about how and when the wages will be paid. Remember that an employer must withhold and pay Social Security taxes. Some families have a bookkeeper who takes care of the checks, the household expenses, and the quarterly reporting. One advantage to using an agency, which I discuss later in the chapter, is that it will take care of the business side of employing people.

Pay can range from the minimum wage (the federally mandated minimum is now $5.15 per hour, but states can choose a higher level) to $20.00

per hour, depending on the area where you live. Many old people are not up-to-date about wages. If this is the case in your situation, do not pretend in front of the elder that the helper will be paid $3.00 an hour and then secretly promise to supplement that amount from your own pocket. The truth will always come out. The purpose of care is not to shield old people from the world but rather to include them in it.

QUALITIES OF A GOOD HOME ATTENDANT

Caregiving is intimate work. Often caregivers are people who want more intimate contact with others. When Victoria Howard and I first started Dana Home Care, many evenings we would walk around our neighborhood talking and glancing into people's windows. People who left their curtains open always seemed more generous to us, more willing to share brief flashes of their lives with people on the street. When I think back to those times, I realize that Vicky and I were longing to go deeper into life, to be more connected.

Another quality that a good caregiver needs is a willingness to work with emotional states as they arise. Many caregivers come from backgrounds where they were criticized or hurt in some way, so they can empathize with the suffering of the frail. But the caregiver must be able to separate her own pain from the distress of the elder. Otherwise, she might take care of old people as a way of trying to fix another's life and thereby avoid her own. Caregivers have to be willing to face the vicissitudes of another's life without rushing to try to make it better. Many caregivers work from an inner need to help people, but most old people don't want to be the victims of a do-gooder. At the very least, the caregiver should be trained to give personal care.

Like old people, who are sojourners on this planet about to take an unknown journey, caregivers are often at some crossroads themselves, taking time out from the regular course of their lives to study, to meditate, to create something artistic. Maybe they are housewives, raising their children, who need a little extra money. Or maybe their children have left home and they are wondering what to do next.

The awareness of being at a crossroads is beneficial in a caregiver. The quality of not-knowing might create a little anxiety, but it also brings the gentleness, courage, and sense of humor required to venture into unknown situations. Good caregivers are willing to feel their way into an elder's life.

Caregivers need to be loyal, forthright, and not overbearing or pretentious. They must have a high tolerance for boredom. The qualities of a good caretaker are beautifully depicted by Tolstoy in *The Death of Ivan Illich*, in the character of the servant who comforts the dying Ivan Illich. He doesn't pretend that Ivan isn't dying, and he goes about providing comfort in a very practical and intimate way.

Live-In Care

Besides caregivers who work by the hour, there are those who live in, receiving room, board, and a salary as compensation. Live-in care is a good solution in certain cases, if an appropriate person can be found. This is usually someone who is doing something else part-time and needs a place to live and a small salary. The live-in is on duty during the night to provide continuity and friendliness. Other helpers work by the hour to do housework, personal care, and other tasks. If the live-in helper shops, cooks a meal, and helps the elder to get ready for bed, that is plenty. You should not ask much more in the way of housework or physical care.

If the live-in person is given clear guidelines about when he is required to be on duty and is given his own space, adequate pay, and family support, this kind of caregiving relationship can be long-lasting and beneficial to both the elder and the helper.

In the early days of Dana Home Care, I lived with an old woman for nearly two years. She was very frail, and I needed the work. I gave her breakfast at seven o'clock, then left for work at eight. After breakfast she rested, then a helper came from ten to one to get her dressed and cook and serve lunch. In the afternoon she sat quietly sorting her papers and listening to music. Some afternoons a woman came to clean house or weed the garden. I got home at five and gave her tea and then dinner. She usually went to bed at eight. I sometimes went out in the evening, but I returned by ten or eleven. If she needed to go to the bathroom in the night, I would get up and help her, but she usually could manage on her own.

Sometimes people hesitate to live in because they're afraid they won't have time for their own lives. But with support and clear guidelines, these kinds of issues can be worked out. Good live-in care can be economical, but it takes a coordinated effort. Frequent meetings and get-togethers with the family should be scheduled to foster communication and support. This will help to keep the atmosphere light.

If money is not a problem, you can hire a professional live-in who works twenty-four hours a day, five or six days a week. Though expensive, these professionals can provide excellent service. Some are paid daily or weekly rates that are less costly than hourly care. Although many people can't work around the clock and still remain cheerful, there are those who can. A professional live-in could be the core of a care team, perhaps consisting of one other main person on the weekend.

Generally, it is extremely hard to find a good live-in caregiver unless the situation offers a pleasant living space, friendly relationships, and plenty of free time. Don't consider a live-in unless there is adequate space. As a rule, only desperate people will move into desperate situations. Back in the days when I would ignore the dictates of common sense in a mis-guided attempt to be helpful, I hired a young, emotionally unstable woman to live in with an emotionally unstable old woman who resided in a small studio apartment. The young woman ended up taking an over-dose of pills and had to go to the emergency room, so no one was helped.

On the other hand, if you find a somewhat troubled person who has a deep calling for the work and a connection to your loved one, do every-thing you can to foster the caregiving relationship. Sometimes people are only temporarily desperate and can relax when properly appreciated. If the old person has a large house, consider having two or three people live in and coordinate their efforts.

The amount of pay for the live-in will vary according to the area of the country, the amount of time the person is required to be on duty, and the personality and level of confusion of the elder. If the old person is very cranky or difficult, the live-in should have few duties, and many other helpers will be required to fill out the schedule. No one, either family member or helper, should be alone for too long with a very difficult old person.

When a younger person shares a home with an older person, their lives become intertwined. This could be good for everyone, but you must be prepared to deal with the emotional and practical complications that, as in any kind of relationship, are likely to arise. The live-in may need to take time off for various reasons, and the elder may feel abandoned and hurt. The live-in may get strep throat and be unable to work for a while—yet has nowhere else to live. The elder may even take a lover and feel that the live-in is in the way. All of these situations will require time and attention to mediate.

OVERNIGHT CARE

Sometimes, instead of having a live-in, it is better to find two or three people to take turns spending the night with the elder. Overnight care is much less complicated than live-in care. Some people will stay overnight for a flat rate rather than an hourly charge. Overnight rates are based on the assumption that helpers will give a little assistance and reassurance and then get a reasonably good night's sleep. When a helper has to be up several times a night, an hourly rate is required.

A good caretaker will try to help the elder sleep soundly. If a nighttime helper has been hired at an hourly rate but has done a good job of getting the elder to sleep through the night, she shouldn't be penalized by then having her wages reduced to an overnight rate.

FINDING A GOOD HOME-CARE AGENCY

A good home-care agency is a treasure. Some agencies find helpers, screen them, and send them out to work with little follow-up. But a good agency will establish a personal and ongoing relationship with both the elder and the helpers. It will create a plan of care for the elder and be flexible enough to adjust that plan in response to the flow of circumstances in a person's life.

When you are selecting a home-care agency, consider the following issues:

- Will the agency come to your house for an initial assessment?
- Is the staff trained?

- Does the agency provide ongoing training, supervision, and support for the staff?
- Does the agency guarantee to send someone to work at the time that you request?
- If the staff person does not show up for work, will the agency be responsible for sending a qualified replacement?
- If it sends someone else, will the agency orient the new person?
- Is there a way to reach the office of the home-care agency twenty-four hours a day, seven days a week, in case of emergency?
- Will there be an ongoing relationship with the agency, and will it conduct a periodic reassessment of the elder's needs?
- Will the agency coordinate the care, or does the agency expect you to do it?

Of course, it would be best if the answers to these questions were all yes, but that will seldom be the case. If the agency provides most of these services and you feel that its staff members care, the agency is worth a try. If the agency does not meet these standards, then you will have to do more work yourself, or you will need a professional care manager.

CHAPTER 3

———◄o►———

The Nuts and Bolts of Daily Care

NOW THAT YOU'VE FOUND HELP, the next step is to consider the other basic components of a circle of care: finances, medical issues, the house and its safety, personal care, giving bed baths, meal preparation, and housekeeping. These are actually the most straightforward situations to deal with, if you take a systematic approach.

FINANCES

Care of any kind costs money. As soon as possible, determine how the care you choose can be paid for. What resources are available? How much of the monthly or yearly income and savings can be used for care without exhausting these resources?

Money is a delicate subject for most families. First, find out what the care is going to cost. Then sit down with the person who will be paying for it—the elder, a family member, a friend, or a trust officer at the bank.

As explained below, compare the cost of home care with the cost of institutional care. Why do you think home care is preferable? It is important that the person receiving the care be included in this discussion, even if he or she is confused and not in control of the money.

Start by evaluating the resources available for care: income and savings, long-term-care insurance, CDs, IRAs, home-equity conversion, loans, support from friends or relatives, Medicare benefits for acute care, and supplemental insurance. In the past, Medicaid was available primarily to support nursing-home care after a person's resources had been exhausted. Now if you live in a state with a Medicaid waiver program, some of these

Medicaid funds can be used for in-home care, if appropriate. Check with the Area Agency on Aging to see whether your state takes part in the Medicaid waiver program.

Then evaluate the cost of home care over a time period that makes sense for your particular situation. If the elder is terminally ill, his or her doctor may be able to give you a realistic estimate of the time frame for which you should be planning. If the elder is expected to require ongoing care indefinitely, you might want to start by evaluating the cost of home care over a five-year period. There are ways to design and fund a good, cost-efficient care program by coordinating community services with family efforts and paid helpers. Also evaluate the cost of nursing-home care over the same period of time. Then compare the costs of home care versus nursing-home care.

Twenty-four-hour care in a nursing home is less expensive than twenty-four-hour care at home. But most older people do not need twenty-four-hour care except for short periods of time. Following the suggestions in this book might help you avoid exhausting the elder's resources. As you consider all the costs, remember to come back to the bottom line—quality of life. A good quality of life does not have to cost a lot, but regrettably, few sources of funding are willing to pay for it.

MEDICAL NEEDS

Although old age is not a sickness, most frail elders suffer from one or more chronic ailments, along with general disintegration of body function. Good medical care is an essential component of the circle of care. There is, however, a great deal of disagreement about what good medical care for the aged should be.

It is essential to have a primary physician or an alternative health-care provider with whom the older person is happy and with whom you as the caregiver have a good working relationship. It is important to let the doctor know that you are developing a circle of care. Discuss with the doctor the care that you feel can be provided at home. Go through the following medical checklist and record your answers, together with any additional questions that may come up:

- What ailments does the person suffer from?
- What medications are needed? Ask the doctor to make medication schedules as simple as possible. Ask, for example, whether the medication would be just as effective taken twice a day rather than four times a day.
- What diets or special treatments are needed, if any?
- Are any nursing procedures required? If so, ask the doctor to order them through a licensed home health agency, so Medicare will pay for them.
- Does the elder need any special equipment, such as a wheelchair, walker, and/or hospital bed? These items can often be billed to Medicare if a doctor orders them.
- Who from the circle of care will be communicating with the physician? Will it be the elder, a family member, a care coordinator, or a caregiver? Will it be a nurse from an agency?

Among the issues that you will want to discuss with the physician is the use of life-support equipment. Advance planning is essential here. If you are closely related to the person needing care, you may have to make life-or-death decisions for her. Hospitals and nursing homes require a directive to be filed in advance, commonly called a "living will" or a "durable power of attorney for health care." These are written documents to guide care for those who have lost the ability to think or speak for themselves, either temporarily or permanently. The family or other caregivers should address this subject with the elder, if possible. Forms for durable power of attorney and living wills can be obtained from hospitals and Area Agencies on Aging.

There are three different kinds of life-prolonging care to consider: cardiopulmonary resuscitation (CPR), artificial provision of nutrition and fluids (tube feeding), and active treatment to fight disease.

Discuss the following questions with your parent, family member, or client: Do you want heroic and lifesaving procedures to be performed in the hospital or at home? Do you want to face open-heart surgery, organ transplant, or other procedures that have made life extension possible? What are the chances of success? How do you define success? (See the resource guide at the end of the book for sources of information on advance medical directives.) What procedures do you want followed at home in the event of an emergency? It is important to discuss the preceding issues with the elder's doctor as well. The relationship with the doctor is more important than the advance directive.

THE HOUSE AND ITS SAFETY

Begin with an assessment of the physical space. Walk through the house, noting any ideas that occur to you that would make the environment safer or more convenient for the elder. As you go through the following questions, don't forget to consult with the person receiving care. A long walk to the bathroom might seem like a problem to you but not to the person who has been navigating the same hall for forty years. If you feel insecure about this aspect of the assessment, call a physical therapist to come to the house and help you.

Can the elder walk alone, or does he need assistance from a person or a walker? Can she see and hear? Does he cook his own meals? Are there steps to climb, rugs to slip on, pieces of furniture to bump into?

Does she have to walk a long distance to the bathroom? What is the bathing routine? Is there danger of slipping? Would it help to have rails on the tub or shower or a bath stool?

What is the bedtime routine? How many times does he get up at night? Is he confused when he wakes up? If he has a urinal or commode, can he remember to use it?

PERSONAL CARE

Good care of the physical body is essential for promoting well-being and friendship with others. The freshness of a well-kept body brings a more relaxed and fresher state of mind. Like the general environment, the body can be a work of art. It's too bad that the standard for beauty in our society is so narrowly youth-oriented. If we can learn to look with eyes not conditioned by the cultural norm, we will see the beauty of gray hair and soft, wrinkled skin.

Generally, two aspects of personal care have to be balanced—cleanliness and communication. You may have to decide which is more important. Sometimes you need to insist, and sometimes you make a suggestion, then wait for the elder to get the idea. Some old people do not like having young people tell them what to do, and certainly not when to bathe.

If the family can afford it and the elder is agreeable, having an attendant come to the house to give personal care even once or twice a week is a wonderful luxury. A trained nurse is not necessary; any sensitive person can learn to give good personal care. It can be one of the best ways to establish a relationship without having to use many words. There are good books on home nursing and personal care listed in the resource guide in the back of this book. In addition, most visiting-nurse services will come to the home to train the family in giving personal care. In many instances, the cost of training a family member is covered by Medicare. Check with the visiting nurse or other Medicare agency.

Often when someone is going through a life change, perhaps lost in reflection or submerged in depression, he or she will not want to bathe. Janet was depressed and would not respond to any pushing. Janet's daughter and her caregivers repeatedly offered to help her take a shower and even brought out basins of water to the chair where Janet sat. That didn't work, so they asked the visiting nurse to come over for a talk about bathing and hygiene. Still Janet refused to take a bath.

Patience was required. The daughter and her helpers kept trying to gain Janet's trust. They made her environment more pleasant by cleaning and preparing better meals, always taking their cues from Janet. One day, when the daughter went to see her mother, Janet said, "I feel like taking a shower today." Janet showered, dressed, and went out to the beauty salon. She kept this up for a few months and then began to refuse care again. The alternation continued, with Janet always controlling her care. Then one day Janet had to go to the hospital. She called her caregiving friends to come see her. "Thank you, girls, for everything," Janet said, just before she died.

Whether or not to intervene in another's life is an ongoing question. Mostly we have to wait until we're asked and then proceed gently. The hard part about waiting is letting go of our own ideas about how clean we think other people should be. Many frail old people take a full bath once or twice a week and just sponge-bathe between bath times. This is fine.

Some elders are extremely modest and do not want to expose their old, wrinkled bodies to youthful eyes.

GIVING A BED BATH

This method for giving a bed bath was taught to me by Eleanor Kraemer, R.N. The instructions here are for giving a complete bed bath, but caregivers can always adapt these procedures to individual needs. For instance, most elderly people can sit on a stool in the bathtub to be bathed. Some sit on the toilet seat in the bathroom to receive the same type of washing. Ellie always stressed that the purpose of the bath was to improve hygiene, to increase circulation, and to provide refreshment, comfort, and communication.

The first task is to prepare the room and assemble the supplies. You should have everything ready in advance. The room should be warm and protected from drafts, and it should be private. The supplies that you will need include: something to protect the bed, a bath blanket or large towel to cover the person, basin, soap or other cleanser, a table or chair on which to put the basin and soap, a washcloth, one or more towels, deodorant, powder, lotion, comb and brush, robe and/or clothing, and shoes or slippers.

After preparing the room, prepare the person for the bath. Make sure she has voided her bladder before getting started. Begin by putting something under her to protect the bed; cover her with a bath blanket or towel; remove clothing. Make sure the elder is as comfortable and relaxed as possible; the bath should be an enjoyable experience.

Fill the basin with warm water, making sure it is at a comfortable temperature. When giving the bath, proceed in the following order (using one washcloth): face, ears, front part of neck, arms and hands, chest, abdomen, back and back part of neck, thighs and legs, feet (unless they are to be soaked in water), pubic region, buttocks, and anal area. You should make a mitten of the washcloth; if the ends dangle, they will feel cold and uncomfortable to the person being bathed. Work quickly, quietly, smoothly; and wash with firm but gentle pressure. Avoid the appearance of hurry, but if the bath is given too slowly, the elder may become exhausted or chilled. Expose, wash, and dry each part separately and thoroughly, covering the area as soon as you are finished. Make sure not to drip water over the person. Change the water often enough to keep the temperature warm and to be able to rinse adequately. Hand the readied washcloth to the person if she wants to wash any part for herself, such as face or "private areas." It is sometimes nice for someone who is bedridden to put her hands into the water.

In washing feet, you may want to allow the feet to soak, to create the illusion of a tub bath. If the person is able to sit on the edge of the bed, she can dangle her feet in the basin once the rest of the bath is completed. If she is in bed, with the legs flexed at the knee, the feet can be placed in the basin. Then remove the feet from the basin and dry them carefully. Apply lotion to legs and feet as needed. In drying, give special attention to the ears, the skin between the fingers and toes, and the pubic region.

After the back has been bathed and dried, a back rub is often relaxing. The amount of pressure to exert depends upon the person's condition and preference. Lubricating with lotion or powder increases the comfort. And be sure to apply lotion or powder to your own hands first. Then apply lotion or powder to any other part of the body as needed or desired by the elder.

After the bath, help the person put on clothing, clear away the equipment, and comb and brush hair. Men may shave now, if they haven't done so previously. The bath can drain an elder's energy, so it is important to attend to his or her immediate needs, such as offering a drink of water or covering with a blanket or sweater for warmth. Then return all the equipment to its proper place; scour the basin; and hang up wet towels to dry or put them in the laundry.

Especially good products for skin care are available from medical supply stores. I like a kind of spray-on cleanser that contains aloe vera and is particularly good for fragile skin. Unlike soap, it does not irritate the skin and does not have to be rinsed off. There are also ointments that can be used on the skin, especially the bottom, to protect against excessive moisture. There are simple ointments such as A and D that help prevent and treat rashes, too. Baby powder is nice to keep on hand, and there are many powders that have pleasant and soothing flower fragrances, depending on the elder's preferences.

Meal Preparation

Many old people have no say in what they eat; they just eat what is served. Many men have spent their whole lives paying little attention to their food. Many women tell me they are tired of thinking about food. And many younger people want to tell old people what to eat. When I hear a forty-year-old woman telling a ninety-year-old man, "Don't eat caviar; the salt will kill you," I think to myself, "Give me a break!" Good nutrition is important as long as it does not depart radically from the elder's habits and as long as it is not an attempt to tell the person what to eat. Involve the elder in choosing menus and mealtimes. Try to follow a doctor-recommended diet as closely as possible, but don't worry too much. Old people, like the rest of us, eat what they want.

Here are some sample menus:

Breakfast:

1	2	3
Blueberries with yogurt and honey	Papaya	Strawberries and yogurt
Oatmeal	French toast	Poached egg on toast
Orange juice	Tea	Cranberry juice

Lunch:

1	2	3
Grilled cheese sandwich	Chicken soup	Broccoli quiche
Asparagus	Crackers with cheese	Fresh fruit salad
Raspberry sherbet	Canned apricots	

Supper:

1	2	3
Chicken	Filet of sole	Chicken
Baked acorn squash	Green salad	Dressing
Green beans	Broccoli	Asparagus
Vanilla ice cream	Rice	Carrots
	Cookie and straw-	Whipped Jell-O
	berry ice cream	

HOUSEKEEPING

Good housekeeping is being mindful of our surroundings and keeping them clean and neat. But it shouldn't become an obsession. Caring for the elder is the main point here, not rearranging his or her life to suit our ideas of order or hygiene.

The drawers, cupboards, closets, and refrigerator should be tidy and well organized—from the elder's standpoint. An old person's home, especially one that has been lived in for a long time, is different from the space of younger people. All the objects in an elder's world have been arranged, over time, according to the perspective of someone who has become stooped, slow-moving, and short of sight. She will be more interested in how the bottom shelf of the refrigerator looks than the top. He needs to know that the butter is on the second shelf on the right. Arthritic hands can get an egg more easily from the door shelf than from an unopened box.

Nothing can drive an old person crazy like having a helper come into his home and rearrange it. I'll never forget a young woman whom I hired twenty years ago to work for an elderly man whose wife had recently died. She had only been working for a couple of days when the man called me and asked if he had to have help. When I went to his house to find out what was wrong, he told me that his helper had rearranged his living room furniture in the night, after he had gone to bed. When I spoke to the caregiver, she told me that the living room looked more attractive the way she had fixed it. I was speechless that this young woman could so thoroughly disrespect an elder's environment. But it turned out that no matter how much training this young woman was given, she couldn't learn to appreciate another's view. She didn't have a knack for taking care.

Caregivers should know where the silverware, cups, and cleansers go and where the towels are kept. They should also be aware that many older people consider it dangerous to allow a burner on an electric stove to become red-hot. These details should be respected. Sometimes changes can be made, but gradually. Communication and respect are the main considerations. If an elder's desk needs to be tidied, the caregiver can sit at the desk with the elder at her side, going through the papers one by one. It will take time, but harmony is more important than efficiency. Later, after communication and trust have been established, efficiency can play a greater part.

Of course, sometimes interventions are needed. I remember an old woman named Mattie, who, after the death of her parents and sister, had been left alone in a large house. As she grew frailer, she spent most of her time sitting in a large chair, eating oranges and bananas, and throwing the peelings on the floor. Her house, with its fourteen untended cats, was a wreck, and so was she. No one wanted to work for her because of the mess.

In this situation, the gradual approach was inadequate. We had to take Mattie out of her house. We drove her to visit the only person in whom she had confidence—her trust officer at the bank. While she was away, a cleaning service came in. The cats went to the vet. The caregivers had to trust their own intelligence and be willing to face Mattie's distress when she returned home. She eventually came to understand that the helpers cared about her environment because they cared about her, and they were able to progress with the care plan.

Any person who doesn't have to struggle just for food and shelter can have a life that is a work of art. Surfaces can be dusted and polished until they shine. A simple flower arrangement can remedy hopelessness. The kitchen, even if it only has a hot plate, can be kept sparkling clean and be adorned with a little potted ivy or an inexpensive geranium.

I remember one woman who lived in a low-income housing project in New York City. Although her apartment was drab, her son cleaned it and waxed the tile floors until they shone. Then he took a chunk of cheese that had come from the welfare office and made open-faced sandwiches, broiled with slices of tomato. I sat with this mother and son at her kitchen table, feasting on delicious cheese sandwiches. It was spring, and there was a water glass of daffodils on the table. Mahler was playing on the public radio station. Even though twelve years have passed, I vividly remember the well-being that was communicated in that moment.

Sometimes it is too much to tackle a whole house at once. If the windows need washing, the carpet is stained, books and magazines are stacked everywhere, and there are cobwebs in the corners, start with the place that is the focal point of the person's life. Many elders have a chair in which they sit most of the time, usually with a table beside or in front of it. Over time, this spot becomes like a shrine. All the person's precious objects are kept there, sometimes jumbled together with pills and books and canceled checks and half-finished glasses of juice. If a helper can gradually bring order to this sacred spot, often the details of the rest of the house will fall into place. Or it could work the other way: if the rest of the room gets cleaner and shinier, then the elder might relax enough to allow order on his table.

Housekeeping issues can sometimes be a source of conflict between an elder and a caregiver, particularly if they are both women. My grandmother was an angel, but she was a bit of a devil about her house. She believed in scrubbing a kitchen floor on hands and knees. "I just can't get it clean any other way," she insisted. Her younger housekeeper thought it was stupid to spend so much time on the floor, and she wanted to buy a mop. They struggled over mops until one day my grandmother fired her.

As grandmother lost her eyesight, she valued what she could control. She was devoted to her old ways and didn't want to learn new ones. The housekeeper could have used my grandmother's frustration as a reminder to expand her view. "What does that mop mean to this old lady?" she might have asked herself. She could have imagined how the clean linoleum felt under my grandmother's bare feet as she walked across it to make her morning coffee. Once the helper had seen the situation from my grandmother's point of view, she could probably have talked her into buying a new mop. "I love your clean floor," she could have said. "I wish I could scrub it as well as you do, but my back hurts me. Do you think we could get a mop?"

CHAPTER 4

———◄○►———

Building a Team

C ARE IS NOT JUST ONE PERSON doing something for another. The attention has to be on creating an environment in which all the members of the circle take care of one another. To work most effectively together, a circle of caregivers must become a team. It is the task of the care coordinator to foster a spirit of teamwork among helpers, including the family, and also to put in place systems that encourage cooperation and communication. That attitude of caring then spreads to the elder.

Organization is key. Nothing is more disheartening to helpers than a chaotic care situation. If there is no organized system of procedures, even the most well-meaning caregivers will falter, the elder will suffer distress, and a downward spiral of blame and unhappiness will result.

THE CARE BOOK

Good communication is at the heart of a good care system. I suggest using a three-ring loose-leaf notebook as "communication central." The book should contain a copy of the elder's daily schedule and menus for that day. Make a chart showing all visits, medications, treatments, appointments, and activities. Write out all routines of care and relevant phone numbers and emergency procedures. I use a calendar to keep track of who is coming to work each day.

There are various ways to organize pages for daily notes. One method is to simply put each day's date at the top of the page. Then, throughout the day, notes of caregiving events are recorded by time.

February 14, 2000

9:30 AM: Jack ate a good breakfast, took two aspirin.

10:00 AM: Jack had a full bath, soaked teeth.

Another method is to get a weekly day-planner book and a stenographer's notebook. Write out all the appointments and visits in the day planner, and use the stenographer's notebook to keep a running commentary of caregivers' notes. Here are some examples:

4/17 PM—Sally

Up at 3:30 PM. Difficulty swallowing pills, so gave them with yogurt and applesauce. Daughter and a friend came for tea. They had a jolly time. Very alert, good appetite. Large BM. Watched David Copperfield on PBS. To bed at 10:30. Balance and mobility good today, though slow.

4/18 AM—Cary

Got up at 10:00 AM and very energetic. Ate a good breakfast of fruit, yogurt, and soft-boiled egg on toast, then spent the morning reading and listening to music.

4/18 PM—Sally

When I arrived at 1:00 PM, she was reading, and then Nancy, the nurse, came.

4/18—Nancy Jackson, R.N.

I changed the DuoDERM patch on right foot. It's helping; area is less red under there. Also flushed out left ear. May need this more. Got some wax out.   —Nancy

After the nurse left, she ate lunch at 2:00 PM. Then did an impressive round of exercises with the physical therapist: sitting, standing, walking. Verbally responsive. A little agitated after the ear treatment. She chose to have a quiet night to read and then settled down. When I asked her if she was ready to go to bed,

she said, "I'm not sleepy, but I don't feel very alive." Bed at 11:00
PM. Small BMS, x 3.

She awoke at 11:45 PM and was making repetitive motions with her
hand. After half an hour, I went in to her bed, and she tried to
get out of bed, saying she had to get home. Her entire body was
tremoring. I wasn't sure if it was preseizure, TIA, or just the
effort to override her body's sluggishness. She said, "I must get
home so that I can go." After further talk, she indicated that it
was her other house that she wanted to see and that she wasn't
going to stay there; she just had to get there to get away from
all the people and so that she could go. I told her I would tell
her daughter, and she agreed that she was sleepy and needed
to rest. Slept deeply and without restlessness for the rest of
the night.

One method that works very well for communication is to divide notebook paper into three columns. The first column is for recording all medications, treatments, and bowel movements, to avoid duplications or
omissions. When a worker comes on duty, it should be clear if and when
medicines were given. This information will also be helpful when communicating with the doctor, who may need to adjust medications. Visiting
nurses, physical therapists, and other professionals also appreciate knowing what medications and treatments were administered since their last
visit.

The second column is for diet. This is a record of what the elder eats
and drinks each day. When several people are involved with meal preparation, it helps to know what was eaten at each meal. There are many
occasions when the doctor will want this information as well.

The third column in the notebook is for comments and a general record
of what took place on each shift.

March 2, 2000

Medications/Bowel movements	*Diet*	*Comments*
2 aspirin No BM	Corn flakes, banana, tea, milk, toast	Couldn't breathe in the morning, but after the breathing treatment, she felt better.
	Grilled cheese sandwich, raspberry sherbet	Napped this afternoon until 3:00 PM. Her sister visited at 4:00 and stayed for an early supper.
Stool softener	Chicken, asparagus, rice, vanilla ice cream	Took a stool softener before going to bed.

The care coordinator should train caregivers to read the notebook, to record all events, and to sign and date all entries. If the senior is interested in the communication book but is too frail to read it, the helper can read it to her. The care book is for everyone on the team. Its purpose is to share information, not to conceal it.

Orienting New Helpers

Time spent orienting new helpers to the elder's world will save a lot of confusion and upset later on. Start by giving each new caregiver a history of the elder's life—where she lived, her interests, how she adjusted to widowhood or retirement. Discuss what the family thinks she needs in the way of emotional support as well as physical help. Introduce the helper to the care book.

Go through the kitchen and show him where the dishes, silverware, pots and pans, and other utensils are kept. A common complaint of elders is that helpers are careless about putting items back where they belong. Explain any dietary restrictions. Discuss how the table should be set.

If housekeeping is part of caregiving, show the caregiver where cleaning supplies are kept and explain any preferences or idiosyncrasies about the cleaning. Demonstrate laundry routines—not only washing and drying but also folding, ironing, and putting away clean clothes. Make sure the helper understands how to work the machines and how to call the repair service if necessary.

Explain medications procedures: who puts them out and when, and how to record them in the care book. Make sure all medications are clearly labeled. Inform the helper of any visits by health-care professionals. Explain the use of equipment, such as a wheelchair, a walker, or an oxygen tank.

Go over shopping procedures and how the money is to be handled. Some families keep a little purse with petty cash, some have charge accounts, and some have household checkbooks. It is best if one person is accountable for the money.

Inform the caregivers whether they are to bring their own food or eat with the elder, and what foods and drinks they can have. If the caregiver is to stay for a few days, food should be provided. Snacks and drinks should always be available for both caregivers and family members.

Let helpers know that they are expected to dress nicely, in good casual clothes. Wearing sloppy clothes encourages a sloppy approach to the work. Sometimes old people prefer that their women helpers wear skirts and blouses instead of slacks. Some caregivers bring a bag with extra clothing to wear on housecleaning or bath-giving days. Show helpers where to hang their coats, where to put their bags, and where to sleep if they are spending the night.

Another way helpers can express good manners is in forms of address. I like to start out by calling an elder "Mr." or "Mrs." or "Ms." I use first names only if and when the elder requests it. When an older person comes into a room, it is proper for the younger people to briefly stand up. If you are going out together, open the car door for the elder, help him or her into the car, and close the door. Provide assistance with the seat belt if necessary. At a restaurant, make sure that the elder is properly seated and can read the menu. If a person is approached with genuine courtesy, almost any other difficulty can be worked out more easily.

Helpers should not accept gifts from elders, so as to avoid possible misunderstandings later. Helpers also need to know the policy on making personal phone calls and about the inadvisability of inviting their own friends to visit, except in special circumstances.

Because the atmosphere around old people is often lethargic, caregivers might tend to spend a lot of time watching television. If the elder wants a helper to sit down and join her in watching a program, that is appropriate, but helpers should be encouraged to design activities that provide more stimulation and variety than just watching TV. The atmosphere in a circle of care needs to be warm and accommodating, not sleepy or sloppy.

The caretaker must be informed about what to do in an emergency. Should the emergency ambulance service be called? Should the helper sit quietly with the old person to wait for family members or the ambulance? Make sure emergency numbers are clearly noted in the care book.

When you are giving an orientation tour of an old person's home, be aware that the elder may feel that his or her place is being usurped, and proceed with sensitivity. Make sure the elder understands the nature of the caregiving relationship. Sometimes old people treat their caregivers like servants, which can lead to bad feelings. Caregivers are best regarded as extensions of the family. Family members often have to see that helpers receive the support they need.

These are a few of the most basic points of orientation. They are good opportunities to open communication with a helper. There is no need to go into too much detail in the beginning; there will be plenty of opportunity for communication as time goes by, as shown in the following sections.

Team Meetings

Another tool of communication for the caregiving team is the team meeting. Each person on the team should have the chance to bring up any issues that need discussion. The elder should be informed that you are going to have a meeting of the care team and should be asked if he has any concerns that should be addressed. He is not usually invited to attend. This is a delicate issue, as the elder might not like the idea that a meeting is being held to discuss him. Explain that the caregivers need to get together to iron out details in order to improve the care. Keep the meeting moving so that it never lasts more than an hour. Helpers should be paid for their time; it is money well spent.

Meetings can be used to work out details of care, especially when a team is in its beginning stages. One of the most important issues for a caregiving team is division of labor. A chart listing tasks and assigning responsibility for each can be very useful here. Who will be in charge of the kitchen? The bathroom? The laundry? The weekly shopping? Light dusting and vacuuming? A cleaning chart can be a useful tool. Keep in mind that caregivers are not a substitute for a regular weekly housecleaning by a paid housekeeper. Caregivers usually don't have time for heavy cleaning. Ideally, each caregiver will tackle the jobs he or she feels most comfortable with. Everybody will do a better job that way.

Another area of discussion for team meetings is food and clothing. Plan the meals for the day or week. Decide who will shop for the food and who will do each step of meal preparation. At what time should meals be served? Decide on place mats, tablecloth, and napkins. Who will make sure the linen is clean?

Issues that require individual attention or special planning might come up. During the meeting, a caregiver might mention that she saw a sore on the elder's back. It is decided that the elder needs to go to the doctor. Who will make the appointment? When should she go? Will transportation be required? Who will provide it? Can shopping be done on the way back? Will they stop for an ice cream? Who will put the wheelchair into the back of the car? All these details can be decided at a meeting.

Often members of the group have to put their heads together and try to see things from the elder's point of view. The "Telling the Elder's Story" exercise presented in Chapter 1 can be helpful at this time. One caregiver can be assigned to play the role of the elder, speaking in the first person in his or her voice.

For instance, if the staff is disagreeing about how the person should be dressed, the elder could be played standing in front of her closet, saying what she wants to wear and how she feels about having caretakers help her dress: "My name is Gladys. I live in Mobile. My house is white. I like to wear casual clothes because I like to garden and walk. I love flowers. I love the feeling of the sidewalk under my feet. I want my clothes to be blue or green."

After the physical description of the environment, move to relationships: "I don't have many friends, but I do have a neighbor down the street whom I like to walk with. I want to look my best when we get together."

Then try to show the elder's state of mind and the obstacles she might encounter: "When I wear nice clothes, I feel more relaxed. I feel better about myself. But lately I can't think what to wear. Sometimes I want to put on a particular pair of pants, but they're too big."

This style of presentation can be used for any issue—food and how the elder arrived at her present diet or the elder's state of mind at five o'clock in the afternoon. Playacting can loosen people up so they communicate better. It also trains caregivers to see situations more clearly. When a caregiver sees how one person plays an elder, it brings up her own ideas about how she sees the person. When the caregiver is back on the job with the elder, she might be more sympathetic or more skillful.

Other types of team meetings can help bring a staff together. A physical therapist or a nurse can be invited in to lead a special training. This is particularly helpful if there has been a change in the elder's condition so that new skills are needed, such as helping him in and out of a wheelchair. Another type of meeting is the large team meeting, at which family members and staff get together. This type of meeting addresses broad issues of care planning and how to handle emergencies.

INDIVIDUAL MEETINGS

Not all problems have solutions, but warmth and clarity of communication always help to ease a situation. In a team meeting, you might see that a helper is angry or depressed. Sometimes helpers take too much upon themselves, then get burned out and resentful. Sometimes they get over-involved with the person in their care. Maybe the elder is distressed and placing an emotional burden on the helper.

Some helpers spend time on the phone talking to their family and friends and neglect the elder. Some helpers have trouble being part of a team. They might be very warm and friendly to the elder and the family but cold and critical to other team members. Sometimes helpers compete with one another to be the favorite. Caregivers need to be supported by the coordinator and the rest of the team, so look for signs of distress.

When evidence of trouble appears, the coordinator should take the helper out to lunch or tea or set up an individual meeting. Before the meeting, research the problem. Find out how others on the team see this helper, what the elder feels about her, and what family members think. Sometimes there is a team member whom everyone picks on. Try to discover what that caregiver does to draw complaints from the others. Sometimes a helper would benefit from a little boost; sometimes he needs feedback, in a gentle way, to let him know what others are thinking. Sometimes it becomes clear that a helper cannot work as part of a team, but that is rare. Usually, a change of focus or an attempt to understand a person brings more harmony into a group.

RELATIONSHIP BETWEEN THE TEAM AND THE FAMILY

In order for a team to work happily, it is essential that the family support the caregivers and that the caregivers keep the needs of the family in mind. Many family members have mixed feelings toward caregivers. Old issues of guilt, sibling rivalry, and fears of abandonment might be projected onto them. Friendliness can be facilitated by always keeping interactions focused on the care of the elder. When individuals are united behind a single task, personal issues are more easily dealt with.

Caregivers should know when family visits are planned, so food and accommodation can be provided. Family members can unthinkingly create upset by leaving dirty dishes in the sink or expecting caregivers to wait on them. A spirit of camaraderie would be fostered if occasionally the family included helpers in dinners out or parties.

Helpers must also keep in mind the needs of the family. Families have to know how the care is proceeding—whether mother is eating, how she's sleeping, what seems to make her happy or worry her. Caregivers should be careful never to take sides when family factions disagree over the elder's care. Family members often know at a deep level what will bring a greater sense of nourishment to their loved ones, so they can be wonderful resources if you want to understand the elder better.

Paid caregivers must be supportive of a family's needs, too. When a family member has traveled to see an aging parent, he needs rest and a good meal. Some caregivers complain that they are only there to take care of the old person and shouldn't have to take care of the family, too. A family has to be sensitive to how much work a caregiver is doing and not overload her or expect her to be a servant. Family members often want time alone with their parents. A caregiver should know when to step back and when to come forward.

CELEBRATIONS

Caring for an old person can be very humdrum without occasional celebrations. Look for excuses to have a party. Encourage the elder to invite her whole family for a reunion or a holiday. Caregivers can get together and plan the feast. They can find out what the family traditionally likes to eat and then supplement it with some favorites of their own. Birthday parties for all members of the caregiving team are great opportunities to bring the team together for fun. The joy of planning and preparing for a party chases away the tiredness that comes from caretaking. Uplifted spirits can carry people through untold difficulty.

CHAPTER 5

―――――◆◦▸―――――

The Daily Schedule

E ACH DAY CAN BE a new page in the book of life, but many old people, especially those who suffer from short-term memory loss, wake up deflated, with no sense of prospects for the day. Elder and helper often share a feeling of uncertainty, wondering how they will make it through the day. The solution is to build a world for the elder by breaking up the day into manageable segments of practicality and celebration.

Sit down with the elder and draw up a daily schedule each morning. Write everything down: breakfast, medicine, personal care, getting dressed, drinking tea, going shopping, resting, and reading. Communicate the schedule to the elder whenever you think she's ready: "This is Wednesday. Would you like a pink grapefruit for breakfast? You're going to have breakfast from eight to nine. Then you usually read and have a short rest. This afternoon you have an appointment at the hairdresser, then your sister is coming for tea at 4:30. After supper, we'll be going for a short drive to watch the swans at sunset. Later, you have that good movie to watch."

Too often the day drifts, so it helps to mark the boundaries between activities. For instance, a caregiver could say, "Now that you've finished your breakfast, would you like to listen to Bach for a few minutes before you get dressed?" That statement acknowledges the end of one activity and provides transition into the next. It also offers a choice. "No, I'd better get dressed now," the elder might say. With this approach, both elder and helper feel a sense of forward movement in life rather than a drifting in boundless space.

A disciplined life is enjoyable, no matter how frail a person is. It feels good to get dressed in nice clothes, to sit down and celebrate with a glass of juice before going in search of fresh vegetables, to find out who did it in a good mystery novel, or to sip a thimbleful of sherry and contemplate a line from Rilke. A morning coffee break, teatime, and cocktail hour turn an ordinary day into a series of occasions. The point is to use basic routines of daily living as a means to support the elder's feeling of being present in the world and to provide stimulation, communication, and a sense of well-being.

Example of a Daily Care Plan

May 4, 2000

9:00 to 10:00 AM	Get up, take a bath, and get dressed.
10:00 to 11:00	Take morning pills, drink tea, and eat breakfast.
11:00 to 11:30	Read and contemplate.
11:30 to 12:00 N	Go to the grocery store.
12:00 to 12:45 PM	Rest.
12:45 to 1:30	Have tea and listen to music.
1:30 to 2:30	Eat lunch and listen to music.
2:30 to 3:00	Get ready to go to the hairdresser.
3:00 to 4:00	Go to the hairdresser.
4:00 to 5:30	Sister coming for tea.
5:30 to 6:30	Go to the park to watch the swans in the pond.
6:30 to 7:00	Drink a glass of sherry and have some cheese and crackers.
7:00 to 8:00	Eat supper.
8:00 to 8:30	Help wash supper dishes.
8:30 to 10:30	Watch video: *The Age of Innocence*.
10:30 to 11:00	Take evening medication and get ready for bed.

11:00 to 12:00 M Read until bedtime.

12:00 M Go to bed.

Morning Routines

Many elderly people wake up in the morning and are not sure where they are. It takes a while for the mind to fully reinhabit the body. Especially when the elder experiences memory loss, most early-morning routines involve helping him or her become more present in the body.

I know an old woman who wakes up in the same bed she has slept in for more than forty years. She opens her eyes and looks around uncertainly. "This is a nice hotel," she says. After her morning routine—robe, slippers, brushing teeth, slow walk to her chair, cup of tea, pills, and breakfast—she is usually back in the present and ready to face the day. She has located herself in her world.

The care schedule has to do more than just fill time with daily routines. It can become a disciplined approach to life that enriches the day rather than drawing attention to despair. The rhythm of daily existence and appreciation of the details of home environment, personal appearance, and food become a way to savor life. Over time, this attention to detail strengthens the elder's sense of place.

Dressing

We express who we are by how we dress. The family and helpers should spend some time going through the elder's closet. Pick out favorite clothes, styles that still work, and preferred colors and fabrics. Repair items that need hemming or mending, and then supplement the wardrobe with new clothes. The person may have lost weight and need a smaller size. If she has become bent or stooped, a different style might be more becoming. Sometimes different shades of favorite colors look better with white hair and aging skin.

Looking at catalogues with an old person is a good project. Shopping is a pleasant outing, if the person is able. Caregivers often take their clients

to shopping malls in wheelchairs to save energy. Some stores will let helpers bring home clothes on approval so the elder can try them on there.

Frail people need clothing of sturdy fabrics that stand up under frequent
laundering, but the fabrics must be soft, for tender skin. An elder should
not wear clothes more than once or twice before they are laundered. Clean,
fresh clothes feel good, and what feels good enhances well-being.

Sometimes caregivers fall into the elder's habitual ways and can see no
other approach to doing things. I once cared for an old man who got himself up every morning, put on his slippers and robe, then walked out to
the living room to watch the morning news and wait for his helper, who
came at 8:00. Slippers were a big issue with this man. He had a spot marked
on the rug where the slippers were to be placed at night. In the morning,
when he swung his legs out of bed, his feet would land on the slippers.
But as the old man's arthritis worsened, he couldn't bend over to use the
shoehorn to get his slippers on. He would have needed an extra hour of
caregiving each day just to help him with his house shoes. His care team
went crazy shopping for slippers that wouldn't require a shoehorn.

Finally, at a team meeting, the supervisor asked, "Why can't he walk
barefoot?" It was such a simple question, but it released team members
from their narrow view. They saw that they had fallen into the old man's
habits right along with him.

Of course, the solution brought up new problems. They had to convince
the man to let the evening helper put bed socks on him, so his feet wouldn't
get cold in the morning, and convince him that he could wait to put on
his slippers. They had to help him practice walking in stocking feet. The
support this elder needed concerning this one issue provided days of good
stimulation and communication.

AFTERNOON ROUTINES

Afternoon routines can be ways to bring more joy, humor, and friendship
into a person's life. They are a good place to introduce stimulating activities and vary routines. When old people become ever more opinionated
and attached to their patterns, helpers can inject notes of elegance, awareness, and fun. After the morning activities of dressing, perhaps keeping
house, and eating lunch, afternoons can be a time for going out into the
world. (See "Other Activities," later in this chapter.)

For many elders, on the other hand, late afternoon and early evening is the most difficult time of the day. As the light diminishes, energy falls, and the person's spirits droop. Our task is to help the spirits rise. Without support during this transition, the elder may sink into depression or become restless and confused.

Often it doesn't take much. When Elizabeth, who had a broken hip, was restless in the late afternoon, she would imagine that little men were coming down the chimney into her living room. All it took to help her relax was to move her wheelchair over to the open front door. She would sit there and watch the college students who lived in her neighborhood as they returned home from school. Watching the young people helped her feel more connected to the world, and her restlessness would ease.

Some elders like to go for drives at this time of day or watch a news report on television or have a glass of juice or sherry with crackers and cheese. If no one is available to share the drink, listening to music might provide companionship. Some people enjoy helping with the preparation of dinner, perhaps snapping green beans or making a salad.

The evening meal can be an occasion for nourishment of the mind as well as the body. When Elizabeth became angry and confused, her daughter would go into the kitchen to cook. Elizabeth had bad teeth, so her daughter often made a meatloaf. She would mix it up in the kitchen, then take it to her mother to ask for advice. Elizabeth would peer into the bowl and say, "It looks fine."

Elizabeth would sit in the dining room while her daughter set the table. She could smell the meatloaf cooking while she drank the glass of wine the doctor had prescribed and watched her daughter polish the silver. After dinner, Elizabeth would be clear and cheerful.

Include the elder in the evening routines of food preparation, serving, eating, and cleanup. Ask her to help with decisions about what to eat. Even if the elder is not coherent, ask her to choose between one food and another: "Would you rather have fish or chicken?" Don't accept an answer like "I don't care. Anything will do." Persist in finding out what the elder likes to eat and how she likes it cooked. Engage her in the process of food preparation in any way possible.

Every meal can be a celebration. Good food attractively presented is healing. It doesn't have to be fancy. A simple omelet with a garnish of parsley makes a lovely meal. Serve it on a china plate with a glass of cranberry juice. The colors, textures, contrasts of temperature, and aroma combine to awaken the elder out of his daydream for a moment.

EVENING AND OVERNIGHT ROUTINES

Watching a video after supper is enjoyable for some old people and their helpers. Let the elder choose what to see. Offer refreshments. But don't just turn on the VCR and leave the room. It's more fun if two people watch together. Talk about the film afterward. My father was crazy about John Wayne movies. Other people might like nature films or historical dramas. Find out what uplifts someone's spirits.

Assess the whole nighttime environment of care. Make sure the bed, the bedding, and the temperature in the room are comfortable. Good evening routines help with sleep: supper at a regular hour followed by a walk or a drive and a regular time to read, watch TV, or visit with a friend. If supper was early or small, a bedtime snack might be welcome.

Darkness throws us back on ourselves in a way that can be frightening. Have you ever awakened from a deep sleep and been unable to remember where you were? Sometimes people get lost in a dream and cannot distinguish the dream from reality. Many older people experience hallucinations. It helps not to struggle with mild disorientation and dreamy states of mind.

At night, the minds of helper and helped may seem to merge. The stream of being of who we are is not so solid in the dark or in the slight confusion of being half asleep. Our awareness extends beyond the body, out into the atmosphere. Communication becomes more simple and effective. Sometimes it's hard to know whether two people are talking to each other or whether the environment is speaking.

For a time, I spent the night with Lane, who had a big bell like the ones schoolteachers used to use. But usually she didn't have to ring the bell; my intuition woke me up. I'd go to her bedside, where I'd slip the plastic bedpan under her bony hips. As Lane sat on the side of her bed, taking pills and contemplating the rest of the night, she would say, "Thank you, sweetie. I don't know what I would do without you." Many times I didn't actually hear her; I'd have fallen back to sleep. Our communication was in the air we mutually breathed.

Old people require sleep at night, and so do their helpers. The need to urinate frequently or sleeplessness due to anxiety or pain are common causes of nighttime distress. Many old people who go to sleep early wake up in the middle of the night. Maybe their medication has worn off. After that first deep sleep, people often doze fitfully until daylight.

If nighttime disturbances are a concern, first consult a health practitioner to see whether there are physical complications. If the elder is having a problem with frequent urination, consult a urologist to determine whether there is any pathology that might be treatable. Ask to have medications checked to see whether combinations of drugs could be causing complications.

Sometimes the best way to manage nighttime toilet needs is a bedside commode. This is a portable chair with arms and a toilet seat. Medical supply stores rent or sell them. If the person can make it to the bathroom, toilet extenders or bars by the side of the toilet help. Some people wear adult diapers at night with extra waterproof pads on the bed.

You might want to hire someone to assist you for several nights when disturbances begin or ask a friend to come along to help solve logistical difficulties. Ethel was troubled by a painful urinary frequency at night. She also was upset that she had to wake up her nighttime helper. The doctor could find no problem, but after Ethel urinated, she had to pour cold water over herself to make the pain go away. The young woman who lived with Ethel worked out a method with a bedpan and a thermos of cold water that Ethel could do by herself. Ethel was relieved not to have to call for help in the night, and you can imagine how happy her overnight helper was to be able to sleep undisturbed.

You might want to invest in an electronic monitor or intercom that allows you to hear what's happening in another room. Even a whisper for help can be detected. You can find these devices in stores that sell medical or baby supplies.

Other Activities

Housework and Deskwork

After my mother suddenly died of a heart attack, my father fell in love and remarried. His second wife, Eleanor, made him take part in domestic chores, something he had never done before. He had to run the vacuum cleaner, take out the garbage, and grocery-shop with her on Saturday mornings. For him it wasn't a burden; it was a way of connecting with his wife and their life together. Involving elders in household tasks lets them feel independent and vital.

Old people who worked outside the home all their lives may be more interested in deskwork than in domestic activities. Decreasing energy often leads to a desk piled up with matters that need attention.

Some elders find it easier to communicate with family members or other helpers about business matters than about personal care. Then again, some people are frightened that their children will steal their money and put them in institutions, so communication about business matters can be delicate. A family member, secretary, or care coordinator can be helpful in scheduling appointments, paying bills, and filing insurance forms.

Going Out

Taking an old person out for a drive or for an appointment or shopping can be a challenge. It helps to be prepared for contingencies. The goal is to reduce isolation by helping the elder connect to a sense of her place within the larger community. Attention to details will help make the outing go smoothly. Where should the car be parked? Who will call the taxi? Will a wheelchair or walker be needed to help the elder get from the car into the building?

If the elder is going for a doctor's appointment, who will communicate with the receptionist? Will the caregiver go into the treatment room, or will she wait in the reception area? To whom will the doctor communicate treatment plans? It is best if the elder and doctor can communicate directly, but sometimes it helps to have a caregiver along to listen and take notes.

Consider preparing a bag to bring along on outings. The bag might contain bottled water, medications, sanitary pads and wipes, sunglasses, cookies, and maybe a book or magazine. If an elder has to wait in the reception area for an extended period of time, he might become agitated, so it helps to have reading material.

The return trip from a doctor's appointment might be a good time to stop for some fun before going home. The more people and events that can be included in the outing, the more it will connect the elder to a broader experience of life. Fill up the gas tank, stop for an ice cream, drive around to look at new houses being built in the neighborhood.

Inviting Visitors

Afternoon is often a good time to invite a friend over for tea. There are usually old friends and neighbors who would like to visit an elderly person. Friends may have fallen out of the habit of visiting because of uncertainty about whether their visit would be a help or a burden. If the elder is confused, the friend may not know how to relate to the confusion and feel uncomfortable.

The way to proceed is to invite an old friend, prepare some tea and cookies, and then join the visit yourself. Do everything you can to make it a pleasant experience for both the elder and the guest. Some elders, in their confusion, have driven away their friends. They may live in isolation because of the fear and grief of saying good-bye, so you may have to help them shift their focus to the hello that precedes every good-bye.

Pay special attention to the welcome. Put a small bouquet of flowers in the guest's bedroom if the person will be spending the night. Or put flowers on the table if the person is coming for tea. Get a cake. Help a visitor hang up her coat. Make the atmosphere of welcome more extravagant than the elder could manage on her own. Frail people really appreciate it when their relatives and friends are properly attended to. As the visit proceeds, helpers can foster good communication and enjoyment. Sometimes the elder wants time alone with her friend, but just as often she will appreciate someone else helping with the conversation.

Pay attention as well to the leave-taking. Help the elder walk to the door to say good-bye. If the visitor has been there for a couple of days, have a good-bye celebration. Help arrange transportation, if needed. Then, allow space for whatever grieving may be necessary. We are always saying good-bye to one part of our life and hello to another, but we often forget to mark the moment.

Friends and relatives will come more frequently if they know that their visits are welcome and helpful. Spending extra time on the details of the visit in the beginning will pay off in more visits, and subsequent visits won't require so much attention to details. When guests feel welcome, they will take care of themselves and the elder whom they have come to see. In one case, a caregiver of a Jewish woman decided to invite the elder's grandson and his family to a traditional Friday night meal. This quickly became a weekly ritual, the high point of the elder's week, and created long-lasting friendships between the family and a series of Friday night caregivers.

WELCOMING MISHAPS

Comforting as daily schedules can be, many elders are stuck in excessive routine. The task then for the helpers is to lighten the atmosphere that surrounds the routine. It sometimes happens inadvertently. In a moment of surprise, an opening is created in which a little freshness can enter. It might feel a bit disturbing, but the dust will settle, and both you and the elder will be energized.

I was once visiting an old woman who had been rude and cranky all morning. Around noon a visiting nurse came to check on her medication. The old woman stared at the nurse's large breasts and asked, "Do you wear a brassiere?" "Yes," the nurse answered, "unless I want to trip." The old woman laughed. In a moment of warm, feminine camaraderie, the elder's spirits lifted, and so did mine. The rest of the day was enjoyable. Stimulation can help bring a person to her senses.

I remember another day when I was taking care of a man who did not want me in his house. He didn't know me well, nor did he want to. He kept shouting, "Can't I get some help around here?" Nothing that I did seemed to be helpful, and the day was dragging on. I asked him if he would like to have a fire in the fireplace, and he agreed rather sourly. I laid some logs in the hearth and lit them. The flames leaped up, and smoke poured out. I had forgotten to open the damper. The smoke set off a deafening fire alarm. The old man was wringing his hands, the dog was barking wildly, and within a couple of minutes, two fire trucks and a police car pulled up.

Although no damage was done, I thought to myself that this would be the last straw with this fellow. In fact, the chaos had the opposite effect. He relaxed and cheered up. He went around to meet each firefighter, saying, "I'm glad our fire department is on the job." He spent a peaceful afternoon and evening reading in front of the fire that we eventually built.

CARE STUDY

Discipline as a Way of Life

———◄○►———

In the twenty years since her retirement from teaching school, Edith had become overly attached to her routines of daily living. As her energy waned, the details of her existence took all her time to accomplish. Edith's doctor said she should go to a nursing home because she had become senile, but Edith didn't want to leave her own home. The task for her caregivers was to enter into her world, not to make changes but to help Edith live her preferred lifestyle.

The helpers attended to the details of Edith's routines as a way to make friends with her. Her activities became the working basis of the relationship. Edith's family and the caregivers accepted her life as it was, made it as good as it could be, and stuck with her to the end.

"I lived my life by my principles," she would say. Never violating her schedule, Edith awoke each morning at 8:30, sipped prune juice, and said her morning prayers. Then she would slowly walk to breakfast, where she used her magnifying glass to read philosophy while she chewed each bite of her morning meat loaf fifty times.

While Edith ate, the helper prepared her food for the rest of the day. She cooked cereal, chopped nuts for Jell-O, and steamed the vegetables that were stored in jars in the refrigerator. Edith occasionally looked up from her book to tell the young woman how to cook the vegetables. "Make them nice and soft," she would say.

The table where Edith ate was full of her projects: scraps of paper with poems, astrology charts, pencils, rubber bands, and books. Bits of food stuck to the plastic cloth. Five fading roses floated in a bowl of water.

Edith's children had scattered, and she wondered if she had driven them away. She had lived in Kansas through the dust bowl days and had seen her life blown away many times. She claimed that her husband had abused her children while she, trying to make ends meet, was working as a schoolteacher. Although Edith's children remembered the story differently, it was true that Edith's husband had left her with children to raise.

After breakfast Edith went into the bathroom for an hour for her morning ablutions. Then she slowly walked to the bedroom to put on her clothes. The caretaker helped her dress, checking each item of clothing for spots. All during the morning routine, Edith would instruct her helper about how to be clean, describing the importance of using one washcloth for the upper part of the body and another cloth for the lower part and where to hang each cloth.

Edith was always teaching her helpers. There was a meaning to each item of clothing that she selected: her red pantsuit for a gray day; a flowered blouse with her tan suit, to remind her of spring. She also taught her helper the proper way to make her bed. Edith lay on the bed to make sure that the blankets came to the right place on her chin before her helper pinned them in place with large safety pins.

This was a world in which the activity of daily living was all-important. Some people focus on relationships, some people live in their minds, but Edith's strength came from her home and from a daily schedule of living honed through many years of practice.

Each activity had a purpose. Edith had little cushions in different chairs to bring comfort when she sat in a particular position. At each meal, she ate a different food. She ate "breakfast like a king and supper like a pauper."

Each time of day brought an activity appropriate for her level of energy. Morning was domestic, the afternoon was for projects, and in the evening she watched educational television or talked on the phone. Caring for Edith meant tuning in to the details of her world. Her relationship with the sacred elements of her life was as profound as that of two lovers dancing in the moonlight.

But taking care of Edith was not romantic work. Relating with her meant working with conflicting emotions. Edith liked to goad people. When she was not sure what to say, she trotted out crusty old beliefs and opinions. Although Edith was dear and likable, her helpers were reluctant to spend time with her, fearing that one violation of her schedule might tear a carefully constructed fabric, and the pain and loss of her life would pour out. Edith, her family, and their helpers faced one another like aliens across a divide. They needed help to relax and start simply relating with one another.

One morning I went to see Edith. She sat at her table eating breakfast and reading, while a helper was busily scrubbing the kitchen floor. "I always said I would rather go on welfare than scrub floors," Edith remarked. My anger flared up. I felt the helper's humiliation and Edith's humiliation, and all the bad feelings between generations. For a moment, I wanted to get up and stomp out the door. Instead, I mentally breathed in our mutual pain and breathed out understanding, over and over. When the helper stood up to survey the shining floor, Edith said to her, "Why don't you sit down and have a cup of tea?"

Such was a typical morning with Edith. The caregivers were often overwhelmed both by the amount of detail that needed attention and by their responses to her remarks. But they learned to take their reluctance to relate as a signal to look more closely at the details of Edith's life. Irritation and boredom are relieved by going more thoroughly into the situation at hand.

Edith's daily schedule reveals how her activities supported her disciplined life:

Edith's Schedule

8:30 to 9:00 AM	Wake up, pray, drink prune juice.
9:00 to 10:00	Eat breakfast, read serious literature.
10:00 to 11:00	Personal care, get dressed.
11:00 to 12:00 N	Errands or bookkeeping.
12:00 to 12:15 PM	Walk or do other exercise.
12:15 to 1:30	Rest.
1:30 to 2:00	Eat fruit plate prepared by morning helper.
2:00 to 4:30	Work on papers, write poetry, do projects.
4:30 to 5:00	Eat ice cream prescribed by doctor.
5:00 to 6:00	Water plants, talk to PM caregiver.
6:00 to 6:30	Eat cereal.
6:30 to 6:35	Take one aspirin.
6:35 to 7:00	Talk on phone or sit quietly.
7:00 to 9:00	Watch educational program on television.
9:00 to 9:30	Eat pureed zucchini and prepare for bed.

Edith had care each day from 9:00 AM to noon. She was alone from noon to 5:00 PM. She had a helper from the neighborhood each day from 5:00 to 6:00 and was alone at night, except for the college students who roomed in the basement.

Since Edith received help when she most needed it, she was able to get by on four hours of care a day, even though she was extremely frail and had been diagnosed as senile. The following entries from Edith's care notebook show how carefully Edith had worked out her life. This detailed approach has worked well for many others. Then care is a support for an elder's disciplined way of life.

Edith's Diet

Breakfast:
    Meat loaf, liver, or chicken
    Two servings of vegetables
    Jell-O salad made with nuts and vegetables
Lunch:
    Fruit plate of three or four kinds of fresh fruit
Afternoon snack:
    Bowl of ice cream
Supper:
    Bowl of whole-grain cereal with nuts and honey
Evening snack:
    Bowl of pureed zucchini

Duties for Morning Caregiver

Daily: Prepare fruit plate with one orange peeled, one apple peeled and sliced, one banana, and other fresh fruit, if available. Cover plate with plastic wrap and leave on kitchen counter.

Monday: Make meat loaf.
    Recipe:
    1 pound ground round
    1 cup grated carrot
    ½ cup chopped onion

½ cup chopped celery

1 can mushrooms, chopped

½ cup bread crumbs

1 egg

1 can tomato paste

Mix all ingredients and bake for one hour.

Tuesday: Make Jell-O salad.

Recipe:

To a large package of lemon Jell-O add chopped nuts, grated carrots, and chopped celery. Chill until set and then cut into two-inch squares.

Wednesday: Cook green beans, corn, and peas. Place in jars in refrigerator to be used as needed.

Thursday: Prepare shopping list:

1 pound ground round	1 package lemon Jell-O
1 chicken or 1 pound liver every third week	14 zucchini
	1 box whole-wheat cereal
1 package green beans	1 jar honey
1 package corn	1 box cookies
1 package peas	1 package toilet paper
1 quart ice cream	1 package tea bags
1 bunch carrots	1 quart prune juice
1 package celery	6 oranges
12 onions, yellow	6 apples
1 package walnuts	6 bananas

Friday: Helper puts away groceries after the shopper delivers them.

Daily: While Edith eats her breakfast, clean kitchen and bathroom. Make sure refrigerator is straightened up and clean. Make sure jars of food are clearly labeled. Make sure all dishes and silverware are in their clearly marked areas.

After helping Edith dress, help her make the bed. Edith will lie on the bed to show where to place the blankets so they come to the right place on her chin. Use large safety pins to pin the blankets in place.

In winter check to see if the sidewalks are clear; shovel show, sweep, and put out salt if needed to melt ice. In summer make sure the sidewalks are clean; sweep if necessary.

Check the lawn for any trash, and water on appropriate day. Check the garden for weeds. If weeds are getting out of control, suggest to Edith that she call the young man who does the weeding and mowing.

Duties for Afternoon Helper (5:00 to 6:00 PM)

Spray ferns and water violets. Puree the zucchini and leave in a pan on the stove with one teaspoon of butter on top.

Set the table for breakfast.

Pour a glass of prune juice, cover with plastic wrap, and put in refrigerator on front of second shelf.

Make sure humidifier is filled.

Turn down the bed, checking to make sure blankets are pinned in place. Put a glass of water on the TV tray by the bed.

Heat cereal so it is ready to eat when you leave at 6:00.

Special Projects for All Days

Type Edith's poems; do the gardening; clean the stairs to the basement. Communicate with the roomers; check to make sure their living area is tidy.

Personal Care

Edith does her own daily washing. Make sure she has one clean washcloth on the towel rack for the top part of her body and one washcloth under the sink for the lower part. Make sure the sink and towels are clean.

On Saturday Edith takes a full bath. Make sure the bathroom is extra warm. Light the gas wall heater. Make sure the water is warm. Use some pink bubble bath, which sits on the edge of the tub. Hold Edith's arm and help lower her into the bath so she does not slip. Use the little blue cloth hanging at the end of the tub to wash her back. Leave her alone for ten minutes so she can wash the rest of her body and relax in the hot water. While she is relaxing in the tub, run two clean towels through the dryer to get them warm. Help Edith out of the tub and wrap her in the warm towels. Make sure she is dry and help her into her well-heated bedroom. Help her lie on the bed.

Every other Saturday, Edith has a massage from a therapist. When the masseuse does not come, gently rub her back, legs, and arms with lotion. Use long, gentle strokes and do not apply too much pressure. After the massage, let her rest for twenty or thirty minutes. While she is resting, clean the tub, then help her get dressed. Periodically check all of Edith's clothes for spots and rips. She can no longer see spots on her clothes.

The amount of detail in Edith's life may seem overwhelming. "Why should she eat meat loaf for breakfast?" her daughter wanted to know. "She should eat eggs like a normal person." But after a time, her daughter dropped her idea of what her mother should eat and began to appreciate her mother's uniqueness. She felt happy that finally, after a lifetime spent trying to please others, Edith was eating the way she wanted. So much of caring depends on learning to appreciate differences.

Edith owned her own home, had savings of around $50,000, and received income from her small teaching pension and from renting rooms in her basement. To be able to stay in her own home, it was essential that she manage on the least amount of care possible. She needed twenty-four-hour care for the last six months of her life. Although her care used up all her savings, the cost was much less than it would have been for a nursing home when calculated over the entire four-year period that was involved, and Edith was able to live as she wanted.

Edith, who had lived through the dust bowl and who had herself grown dry and dusty, died on a hot, windswept day in the fall. She had been failing and had been in bed for several days. The young women who helped Edith had moved her bed into the living room, so she would be part of the life of the house. Her helper walked over to check Edith, then she sat back down. Suddenly the door blew open. Edith had died. She seemed to have gone with the gust of wind.

PART TWO

THE SUBTLETIES

————◄o►————

Enriching the Elder's Environment

T HE OTHER DAY a friend remarked that her frail mother was like a plant that blossomed when her spirit was watered and drooped when it wasn't. It's a wonderful image to describe the environment of caring.

Plants synthesize their food from their surroundings, drawing water and nutrients from soil, reaching up for light. Plants make an exchange with the environment, giving oxygen and receiving carbon dioxide. Research shows that plants thrive best not just when they are watered and fed, but when they are nourished with love and attention. Plants are not isolated beings.

Enriching the elder's world is more challenging than caring for plants. A once full life may now have become impoverished, or existing imbalances may have been exacerbated by old age. Enriching the environment can often help. Despite the suffering of human existence, it is possible, in unexpected ways, for the mind to relax and discover the simple, ordinary enjoyment of the moment. Then unbalanced states can be eased, transformed, or seen through.

NOTING IMPOVERISHMENT

I was visiting a nursing home one day as an aide passed out glasses of juice. A social worker watched as the aide handed a glass of tomato juice to a very old woman in a wheelchair. Then the social worker walked to her desk and checked off "sensory stimulation" on her care plan, telling me, "The sharp bite of the tomato juice will stimulate her senses and make her less confused." But the young social worker was so absorbed in her plan that she didn't notice that the old woman had poured the juice on the floor. "I hate tomato juice," she said, to no one in particular.

This kind of inattention can happen at home as well. One day a well-intentioned young man visited his grandmother. "Would you like a dish of yogurt?" he asked her. "I don't like yogurt," the old woman answered. But the young man, in his zeal to help, paid no attention to what she had said. He served her up a dish of yogurt. When his sister asked him why he was giving her yogurt, the brother answered, "She's confused. She forgets what she likes." Picking up her spoon, the grandmother said, "I hate yogurt," then ate it dutifully, taking no pleasure in it.

I was once consulted by a caregiver to help her work with an elder who had started spitting. This old man, who had always had exceptional manners, would wander around his apartment and spit in the corner or behind the sofa or under the table. His caregiver thought that he might be expressing buried anger—expelling something that he was unable to "swallow"—or that perhaps he had something physically wrong with his swallowing mechanism. As the first step, a physical examination was performed, but no physical cause could be found.

Then we looked at the times when the elder did not spit. For instance, he loved to go out for lunch to a deli, where he would eat a hot dog and watch people. When he felt connected to the stream of life, he remembered his dignity, and he didn't spit. We concluded that the spitting was an unconscious signal that he wanted more stimulation. We needed to enrich his environment.

We made trips to the deli a regular event. We also arranged for the man's daughter to come over as often as she could and join him as he watched television. She would sit on one side, the caregiver on the other, both with their arms around him so that their arms crossed over the back of the couch. The old man seemed to feel enfolded and nourished; he relaxed, and the spitting stopped. This brought the daughter and caregivers together as well, so that they, too, could relax better into the situation.

To figure out how to enrich the environment, use your own senses to gather information about the elder. I look for places where the elder's life feels undernourished. First, I locate the person's favorite chair. If there is no favorite chair, maybe she is too scattered or lacks a proper sense of place.

If there is a chair, I sit in it myself and look in all directions at what is in the line of sight. I try to inhabit the skin of the elder. What do I see, hear, touch, and feel while sitting in the chair? Do I look through a window? Do I look at empty white walls or at family pictures, paintings, or objects of interest? Are there sounds from within the building, sounds from the street? Does the phone ring? Can the person hear? What is the texture of the cloth of the chair, the rug on the floor? Do I look at clutter or order? Do I see dirt or cleanliness? Are surfaces dull, or do they shine?

Next I notice the general feeling tone of the elder's atmosphere. Do I feel happy or sad, calm or agitated? Does the energy circulate or feel congested and stagnating? Do I feel claustrophobic or expansive?

Then I take another look at the daily schedule to see how much time the person spends alone. What kind of support does the elder have for being alone? Can he use the telephone? Does she know when someone is coming? Does he have something to read? Can she get a drink of water? If the person spends too much time alone, how can more people be brought in?

I think about the helpers as well. Are they using the activities of daily living as a means to communicate, or are they just trying to get them done as quickly and efficiently as possible? Are they listening to and learning from the elder? Are they mindlessly trying to keep the old person occupied so they can take a break? Do they attend to the details of daily living as a way to help the elder appreciate life? Do they create small segments of activity and rest? Do they work with boundaries by making each activity or period of rest include a beginning, a middle, and an end? When caregiving becomes too regimented and humdrum, attention to enriching the environment can turn the task into a creative endeavor.

ENRICHING THE ELDER'S PHYSICAL ENVIRONMENT

Sometimes when all the sense fields are reduced, the mind takes over, and a person's life becomes too conceptual. Someone who can't see or hear well might tend to live too much in the past. It's commonly assumed that old people lose interest in the environment, but this apparent uninterest is usually a sign of the loss of sensory stimulation. Engaged senses help the mind relax. For all elders, it is important to provide a stimulating environment.

Those who are frail and confused generally have a very small arena in which to live their lives. If the person stays in one room, you have the environment of that one room to work with. Look to see what can be done.

Are shelves needed to organize the space? Is there a chair for a visitor? You can't change the size of the room, but you can work with the sense perceptions: a soft touch, a pleasant sound, the sight of something beautiful. Can the room be made brighter or more colorful? Favorite colors are nourishing to a person's spirit. My grandmother loved green walls to calm herself down and wore red to perk herself up.

I usually ask a person to tell me her favorite colors, but some people feel insecure when they are asked a direct question, as if there were a right or wrong answer. If an elder can't tell me her favorite color, I look in her closet to see the colors of her clothes. I notice the colors of her dishes and towels. You can begin to use the power of color by setting the table with bright place mats and matching napkins, putting flowers in the bedroom or by the elder's chair, and using colored sheets and nightgowns. If you are interested in going further with color, Helen Berliner's book *Enlightened by Design* (listed in the resource guide at the end of this book) provides some excellent suggestions.

Notice the lighting in the person's room or home. Good light lifts the spirits. A room with the play of both light and shadow is more interesting and more beautiful than a room where the lighting is even. Light brings cheerfulness and insight, whereas shadow encourages reflection. Good light draws the energy outward, preventing too much turning inward.

Of course, season and the climate will influence lighting. People who live in dark, cold climates need more light in the winter. People who live in hot, bright climates may need more subdued indoor light.

Fire is a wonderful source of warmth and light. When adequate supervision is available and proper precautions are taken, people who have fireplaces and wood-burning stoves may enjoy watching the flames and feeling the warmth. Candles can also enrich the environment, bringing warmth and light and serenity. Note that too much heat in the environment, especially artificial heat, can dry the skin and eyes as well as the throat and sinuses, sometimes causing a dry cough or headaches. In this case, explore the use of humidifiers, aquariums, and vaporizers. If the air is too moist, dehumidifiers can help.

Lovely objects in the environment spark the attention, lift the spirits, and lend a feeling of celebration. Flowers are an excellent way to beautify the elder's surroundings. They add not only color but also texture, fragrance, and life. Gathering flowers—whether from gardens, fields, or flower shops—delights many people. Flower arranging is an activity that even the most confused person can accomplish with a little assistance. (A note of caution: some people are allergic to flowers.)

The sense of touch is also important in the environment. As people age, the hearing may go, the eyes may fail, but the sense of touch remains. Especially when someone is confused, clothing should be pleasing to the touch. Sheets and pillowcases should be soft. Bedclothes are best in cotton, flannel, or silky fabrics. You don't need to buy something new; many elders prefer their old things to new ones.

How you touch an older person is also important. Many elders have lived without being touched, sometimes for years. Approach the person slowly. A pat on the arm is often better accepted than a full body hug. But don't underestimate the impact of that small gesture. One opportunity to touch people lovingly is during personal care, such as bathing. After the bath, you can smooth on lotion. Massage is helpful for most old people. If finances do not permit regular appointments with a licensed masseuse, or if the elder resists out of fear of intimate contact, there are other ways to touch. When I would help my father put on his sweater, I always smoothed it down his back and patted it into place. When we walked, I took his arm or held his hand.

Another method of touching that is comforting and not too threatening is a foot bath and foot rub. Fill a plastic pan or bucket with warm water. Put newspapers or a cloth on the floor and set the pan on it. Help the elder to soak his feet for as long as the water is comfortable. Then dry the feet, making sure to dry between the toes. Wrap one foot in a towel to keep it warm and massage the other foot with lotion. Be sure to wipe off the excess lotion with a towel and check that the feet are not slippery before the person gets up.

ENRICHING THE ELDER'S STATE OF MIND

What expands the mind so that it feels full and rich? It might be something simple that helps an elder's mind relax—a shared joke, a pet's soft fur, a massage, a steaming cup of coffee, or exercise. It might be recalling a friend or a lost love. It might be simply sitting still and being present with a person.

Smells and tastes stimulate the memory. The smell of a freshly mowed lawn can bring back the memory of another time and place, perhaps happy summer days as a child. Sometimes when one sensory field is not working well, another takes over. My grandmother was nearly blind, but she could hear a pin drop in another room. She could touch her kitchen sink and tell whether it was clean or dirty.

The writer Marcel Proust is known for his ability to describe moments of sensory stimulation, the most famous being when he was ill and his mother brought him a cup of tea and a little cake called a madeleine. "No sooner had the warm liquid mixed with the crumbs touched my palate than a shiver ran through me and I stopped, intent upon the extraordinary thing that was happening to me." He began to remember his aunt who had given him little bites of cake dipped in tea. This opened him to a stream of memories: her house, the town where she lived, and much more. Sensory stimulation can bring up old memories for an elder, too.

The body is a support for the mind. Personal care—wearing nice clothes, eating tasty and nourishing food, and taking good care of the body—can go a long way toward relaxing a person's state of mind. Exercise can be adapted to a level appropriate for the elder: range-of-motion exercise for the very frail, walking, T'ai Chi, dance, and movement therapies. A physical therapist who specializes in working with the elderly can help you find exercises suited to each person's abilities or circumstances.

To enrich a person's life, food needs to be varied and sometimes shared with others. Though elders are often conservative in their eating habits, food can be an excellent way of moving from isolation into a more expanded way of being. Lane ate chicken soup for lunch every day. At first she ate it because she liked it, because she thought it was good for her, and because she was embarrassed to tell her lunchtime helper that she was tired of it. In the end, she ate it because it had become her habit to do so. The woman who made the chicken soup made it because she thought Lane liked it, because she thought it was good for Lane, and because she was afraid to suggest anything new. In the end, she made it because it had become her habit to do so.

One week the woman who made the chicken soup got sick. Another woman came in her place, and the new helper made an omelet. The shock of the change, the courage it took to taste the first bite, the new flavors, perked Lane up. Before long she was eating meatballs and greens and grapefruit and avocado salad.

Stimulation always has to start from the elder's point of view. A woman once asked me why her husband, Dick, seemed so disconnected and confused. During a consultation, I saw that Dick had become an object of care instead of a person. Every morning before he could have a cup of coffee and read the paper, he had to have a bath and get dressed, which took an hour. The care team had become fanatical about cleanliness at the expense of respecting Dick's own biorhythms. Most of his life, Dick had had to arise early to go to work. In his old age, he preferred a slow start to his day. When he was allowed to have breakfast before getting dressed, he perked up.

One reason that Dick was so lethargic in the morning was that he stayed up late at night reading mystery novels and smoking cigarettes. He had reached a point at which reading mysteries and smoking seemed to be his only interests. They helped him ignore his dissatisfaction with being old and retired and unable to express much passion in his life. All the caregiver plots to get Dick to stop smoking and to start walking ended in frustration. A physical therapist walked out on him in disgust. The more Dick was pushed, the more confused he seemed to get.

But even a harmful routine can often be turned into a propeller of good cheer, to fan the flame of life. One day Dick received a form letter in the mail urging the smokers of the city to unite. On his own, he filled out the form and walked to the mailbox to mail it. The helpers saw that if Dick were interested in something, he was willing to walk and could remember things. He just wanted to do things his own way.

The helpers decided to stop judging Dick and to enrich his world with more stimulation and more communication. They bought him easy-to-operate and colorful cigarette lighters and attractive ashtrays. Of course, they made sure that he was exposed to warnings about smoking, reports from the surgeon general, and treatises on how to quit as well. But they also gave him newspaper stories on smokers who wanted to assert their rights. As team members began to work together, they found a cheerfulness that outweighed their aversion to smoking and concern for Dick's health.

Dick's habit sometimes helped provide stimulation in other ways. One day he had to go to the doctor. In the cab, he lit a cigarette, right under the no-smoking sign. "You're not allowed to smoke in this cab, sir," the driver told him. "The hell you say," Dick answered. At that, the cab driver screeched to a halt and made Dick get out in the middle of a busy street. Although the driver might have been a little harsh, Dick did receive good, direct communication. For the rest of the day, he was alert. And on his way back from the doctor, he refrained from lighting up a cigarette.

Sometimes it takes something outrageous to change the atmosphere. Once I helped a daughter take her mother to an awards ceremony. We traveled to another town and stayed in a hotel. Suddenly the mother didn't want to attend the ceremony. "I'm not going," she said. "I'm going to jump out the window and kill myself." The daughter and I looked at each other and with one mind said, "OK, you can jump, but you have to eat your dinner first." We ordered room service, ate dinner, and the old woman relaxed. After dinner we went to the ceremony and had a pleasant time.

If the energy seems stuck, I sometimes try to stir up the atmosphere to make it lighter and freer. Once I faced a long afternoon with a frail old woman who didn't want me to be there with her. She kept asking me, "Don't you want to go?" After an hour of this repeated questioning, my responses were getting stale. Finally, I decided to go with the flow of her energy. I took her by the arm and walked her to the car, saying, "I do want to go, and I want you to go with me."

We headed downtown, where I spotted a town fair. As we walked through the crowds, we smelled hot dogs roasting and were jostled by children carrying cotton candy. The reverberations of rock music from a local band assaulted our ears. Before long the old woman said, "Take me home." She was not confused; she really wanted to go home, and so did

I. We had connected with the juicy confusion of life, and it was a relief to go home and rest.

In order to enrich the elder's state of mind, you need to relax your own. The practice of working with someone old involves learning to calm panic in the midst of confusion. But it is important to realize that even though it goes against the grain, you don't have to calm a person down by throwing a wet blanket on her fire. The stimulation of people, ideas, or breaks in routines can disrupt a pattern of confusion or a stuck emotion, allowing it to settle or pop open and dissolve. The older person's panic and your panic can thus become the catalyst for developing confidence in yourselves and each other.

ENRICHING THE ELDER'S SOCIAL LIFE

If an old person is feeling low, consider organizing more family gatherings, reunions, parties, or dinners. Sometimes families don't get together at the home of a frail elder for fear it will be too much for her to manage or because they don't want to burden caregivers. If an elder suffers from short-term memory loss, family members might assume that visits won't help because she will not remember them. But one family party can do more to enrich the life of an elder than a hundred visits from a nurse or social worker.

Though it is important to entertain at a level the elder feels comfortable with, remember that food and table settings are not the main point. The family can cook or the event can be catered, but the essential point is celebration. The excitement might be a strain on the elder's energy, but there will be plenty of time to rest later. When a person's spirits are lifted, it is easier to rest. I've seen family visits give an elder energy and strength that lasts several months. And the family is strengthened, too. During the family celebration, it's nice to take photographs and collect them in an album. Many old people spend a great deal of time looking at family photos.

Family members often assume that the elder only wants to see the family. While the family is usually the strongest heart connection and source of nourishment, it is good to invite in friends as well.

I know one very elderly woman who moved from her own town to live close to her daughter, leaving behind her old friends. The daughter has worked to facilitate new relationships for her mother. She brings friends to tea who she thinks will be sympathetic to her mother. The caregivers go out of their way to bake cookies and cakes, slice fruit, and make tea. The house is filled with a sense of generosity and abundance and welcoming.

One neighbor, who is a young mother, sometimes visits with her three-year-old son. The old woman and the little boy enjoy each other. The elder's daughter took pictures of her mother and the toddler, so between visits her mother can remember this new presence in her life. The daughter bought small presents for the child, so each time he visits, the elder has something to give him.

Traveling to visit friends and relatives enriches a life. Some day-care programs provide transportation or a sheltered environment for old people who live in the same area to spend time with one another. For these or longer trips, especially, caregivers or family members need to travel with frail elders, and the trips do take careful planning. People who suffer from short-term memory loss can become disoriented while traveling. Taking along familiar personal items and favorite books can help. A sleeping pill or tranquilizer may be needed to help with sleeping in an unfamiliar bed the first night away from home. The benefit of keeping up an elder's connection with family and friends and the fun that goes along with a visit make the travel worthwhile, even if it is temporarily confusing or tiring.

Family celebrations show the caregiving staff the particular ways in which a family finds enjoyment. Then when the family is gone, the helpers can create occasions for the elder according to the familiar style of celebration.

Elizabeth had a young woman, Nancy, who lived with her. While Nancy was at her student-teaching job, I was the daytime helper. Each day when Nancy came home from work, she would have tea with Elizabeth. Sometimes I joined them. Sometimes we would invite a friend of Elizabeth's or a friend of Nancy's or mine. Elizabeth would sit at her dining room table near the window, looking out onto the backyard with its bird feeder and gazebo. Nancy would set the table with handwoven place mats and bring out shortbread cookies from Scotland. While the water boiled, Nancy arranged fresh flowers and put on music. She built a sense of celebration.

At the first tea party, Elizabeth dropped cookies in her tea and made a mess. But before long she began to drink and eat with dignity. She looked forward to these occasions. In her eighty-fourth year, Elizabeth sat with her friends, sipping tea and watching birds bicker with a squirrel while snow fell softly.

————◆◇▶————

CHAPTER 7

Letting Go of the Old,
Accepting the New

I HAVE A FRIEND with a rich aunt who was an invalid all her life. She had two strong beliefs: you shouldn't fraternize with the servants, and drinking alcohol is the devil's work. So you can imagine my friend's shock when she visited her aunt and found her not in bed but in the kitchen, drinking sherry and talking to the cook.

Had my friend's aunt gone crazy? Or had she simply found the wisdom to let go of worn-out patterns and embrace a new way of being? The old woman was taking a new approach to her world, free of her habitual opinions that she was sick, that she didn't drink, and that she would never fraternize with the cook. There is no need to panic when you see unusual behavior in an elder. When old people are abandoned by their former ways of life, they have to find new ones. An important part of our job as caregivers is to help the elder let go of outmoded ways of doing and being—and, if possible, to embrace new ones.

Some elders let go easily. For those who are having difficulty, a nourishing environment can help. Care can be more than trying to patch up the cracks. This chapter explores how you as a family member or caregiver can help the elder adjust to loss by accepting change.

FEELING THE ELDER'S LOSS

Think about how loss feels, from your own experience. You might be going forward with your life when your husband announces that he wants a divorce. Suddenly the earth seems to fall out from under your feet. You have a feeling of sinking and disorientation. Your legs turn to jelly. Then you begin to lose track of the details of your everyday life. The emptiness of loss is hard to stay with. You feel confused, and you try to grasp onto something. You might get angry or feel like giving up in despair. It could take a while before you can find your balance with a new way of being.

When an elder loses the familiar ground of work, mate, or health, he might feel as if he is sinking. As his accustomed self-image falls away, a feeling of heaviness is common. He may want to sit or lie down most of the time. Doing anything feels like too much effort. The digestive system may not work well, so it is hard to digest not only food but new ideas as well. Many vulnerable and lonely old people are plagued by a nagging sense that something is missing. The elder may want to hang on to familiar ways, to the point of feeling paralyzed. When a husband dies, a wife may go on living as a wife instead of entering into a new way of being. A person may be forced into retirement but go on thinking about his business, unable to pursue new interests.

When people have lost some of their social conditioning, anything can happen. Some elders become more cheerful. Some become passive and quiet. Some people become willful and combative. Some are haunted by old desires. Ego cracks, and longing seeps out. Some enter a mystical world, where they see visions of beings from another time and place.

Sometimes when you're just sitting with an old person, you notice that his mind has slipped away from the here and now. He has entered the flames in the fire or become a bug on the ceiling or a child in the distant past. We all get carried away by trains of thought, but when our lives are active, we are soon brought back by some demand—the phone rings, or the light changes to green. Old people, who may not have a ringing phone to bring them back, tend to get lost in their ruminations. Many of the symptoms of the frail elderly, such as failure to recognize familiar faces, have to do with spacing out. Old people often have a hard time getting back into the familiar, concrete feeling of being enclosed within the physical body. The task for the caregiver is to help support their sense of place within the ever-changing flow of events.

Helping the Elder Let Go

People often ask me why we don't just let elders space out and stay there. But even in old age, with its very real suffering, forgetting the body is not recommended. Letting go does not involve going somewhere else. Letting go involves relaxation and release. It happens when body and mind are working together. It is perking up that leads to letting go. Well-being arises by being present with whatever the world has dealt us.

The way to start is to see where the sinking has taken the elder. Listen, observe, and take an interest in his world. That will make him feel nourished and present. Attention to the details of the elder's life is a means of making friends with him. That friendship will help the elder connect with and trust his own inner strength, which, in turn, will help uplift his spirits. Someone who is nourished can see where he needs a helping hand and where he can do things for himself. Eventually, the attitude of attention will surround the old person, and he will be unable to resist it.

To create genuine support, look at the elder as an individual. Ask yourself, How can I help this person be in this moment instead of longing for days gone by? Look to see where the elder in your care finds her home. Does home lie in her relationships with her mate, her grown children, her friends and caregivers? Is home her failing body? Is home in the heart? Maybe home is in the mind. One friend told me that his father, who is losing his eyesight, plans to spend the rest of his life reciting his favorite chapters from the Bible. Silently acknowledge the feeling tone that surrounds the desire. Look at what details make the elder feel more at home. When someone is feeling at home, it is much easier to let go.

Sometimes, instead of creating an environment in which the elder can relax, we keep trying to prop up his basic sense of ego. But propping creates anxiety: there is always the fear that the prop will give way. For instance, the elder doesn't want a stranger to take care of her, and the family buys into her fear. They decide to do the caretaking themselves, with no outside help. Then they become anxious, because they know they have taken on more than they can handle. Or a family member might hire a single caregiver instead of creating a team, so the elder and the family grow dependent on that one person. Even though the situation may be in hand for the moment, there is constant worry about what will happen if the caregiver quits.

One elder couldn't stand seeing two family members talking to each other, fearing what they might be saying about her. The family members propped up her anxiety by not talking to each other. Instead, they could have acknowledged the elder's fear of losing control. They could have told her what they needed to talk about, perhaps including her in the conversation. By not falling into her anxious state of mind, they could gradually have increased the trustworthiness of the environment and supported her ability to let go. Propping a person up is based on not trusting the strength of the elder or yourself. It is like putting a Band-Aid on a big, open wound.

LENDING PHYSICAL AND EMOTIONAL SUPPORT

Alexandra Evans is a caregiver who uses physical means to strengthen psychological well-being. She noticed that one woman for whom she was caring was perching on her sofa with her back hunched. The woman couldn't see and appreciate her world, because she was always looking down. The care team placed cushions around the woman to try and prop her up, but the cushions kept falling on the floor.

Alexandra decided that the woman needed a firmer seat so that she would have a stronger place in the world. She had the sofa rebuilt and recovered. From that new, firm seat, the elder could look up and out at her living room with a straight back and head.

Next Alexandra called a physical therapist, who came and taught the woman the proper way to use her arms and legs for standing and sitting. The frail woman regained a feeling of dignity despite her immobility. The circle of care helped the elder find a good seat, and the seat helped her feel the strength of her own being.

Support means helping people find and appreciate their place in the world. It takes humility and gentleness on the part of the caregiver to promote an elder's self-respect, so that instead of feeling like a burden, he can feel the dignity of his place as the center of the circle of care. Of course, you don't have to rebuild and recover the furniture to support someone. If a person is stooped over, you can kneel down and look up. Once you see the world from her point of view, you will know what needs to be done.

When circulation decreases, the efficiency of internal systems declines, and a person turns inward. There may be decreased oxygen to the brain, swollen ankles, or poor digestion. There may be a stiffening in the joints and muscles. This loss of circulation may appear as an excessive self-absorption and isolation. Emotions can get stirred up. The smallest provocation may spark an angry outburst, perhaps as an unconscious attempt to feel something instead of nothing.

As a person slows down and begins to let go of life, old hurts that have been buried for a lifetime may surface. In that atmosphere, old wounds may reopen for the helpers, too.

We all tend to mix up what happened in the past with what is happening in the present. If an elder tells a helper how to boil an egg, the helper might feel criticized and resistant. Instead of hearing the elder, she's hearing the voice of her mother, who always tried to tell her what to do. Old people do the same thing. I recently saw an elder try to hit a caregiver. As she raised her arm, she called out her sister's name. She was still angry with the sister for a rivalry that happened seventy years ago.

Elders are often hurt if they can't keep up with a conversation or if their son or daughter doesn't call. These hurts frequently manifest themselves as anger and blame. Caregivers, too, can get angry or defensive. It is often impossible to get to the root of emotional distress. The best approach is to let all feelings be, with sympathy but without propping up someone's neurosis. You don't have to agree with a person's resentment, but you can give her a cup of tea and let her rest for a moment until she settles. A supportive circle of care tries to create a sympathetic environment, in which old emotions can finally relax.

ENCOURAGING COMMUNICATION

The fear of emotional outbursts can lead to care that is overcontrolling. Both elders and caregivers become afraid to let life change happen. You might spend weeks or months tiptoeing around, trying to avoid a confrontation. Communication becomes indirect and manipulative. The atmosphere can become heavy with the weight of unexpressed and unresolved conflicts. Before long, everyone in the circle of care begins to feel claustrophobic.

When this happens, helpers need to develop an appreciation for whatever communication is being presented and remain neutral even in a charged emotional situation. Sometimes you can act as a lightning rod, receiving the volatility and letting it escape harmlessly into the ground. One useful form of communication is called purring, in which you respond with sounds: "mmmmm" or "hummmmm," without having to say no or yes. Purring acknowledges the being and desire of the elder without giving in to any insanity. Here are some other suggestions for improving communication.

Trust yourself. Don't be afraid to go with your instincts and be honest. I once cared for an old woman who wanted her daughter to take care of her. Instead, she had me, and she began to feel sorry for herself. Day after day she said, "I'm dying; call my daughter. I'm dying; call my daughter." When the daughter came, the woman changed her request. "I'm dying; call the doctor." I could tell that the woman was not dying. She was attached to seeing herself as a victim of abandonment. She wanted to exert her will, so we would take pity as well as some action.

One day she lay on the sofa with one arm over her eyes. "I'm dying; call my daughter," she told me. "Your daughter can't come today," I replied. "She sent me instead." "Why?" she asked. "Because I work with dying people. Your daughter thought you might like to talk about dying." But this dear old woman did not want to talk about dying. She sat up, walked over to the dining room table, ate a good lunch, and didn't mention the subject again for quite a long time.

One night an old woman wanted to go out for a drive. It was cold, and the roads were slippery. I trusted myself enough to say no, letting go of my desire to please her. Because I trusted myself, she trusted me as well. *No* doesn't have to be a tool of control; it can be a starting point of communication.

Listen to the elder. In old age, it doesn't matter whether someone craves philosophy or too much chocolate, whether the object of desire is good or bad. Listen to the desire being expressed and use it as a way of reaching out to the person.

Once I was part of a care team helping an old woman who lived in a small house by the sea. She had problems with her memory and was often restless. One late spring night, I heard a scratching noise. I came down the stairs and saw her in the living room dressed in her flannel nightgown with a shawl around her shoulders and a fur hat on her head. She was tapping on the door with her walking stick.

My first reaction was to prevent her going out in the cold and dark. I didn't want my sleep interrupted. But some intuition moved me beyond those habitual responses. I called the other caregiver, and the three of us went out into the cloudy night. With a helper on each arm, the elder led us on down a rocky path to the water. Just as we reached the edge of the shore, the clouds parted to reveal the moon, golden and full. We were no longer helpers and helpless but three sojourners in the night. How precious life seemed, as we made our way back up the path to bed. What a gift to have said yes to the spirit of the moment, to have let in the magic of the night.

Look for blocks to communication. Blocks may be the elder's resistance—or the caregiver's. Once a friend and I were taking care of an old woman who was restless and confused. When we finally got her into bed at about eleven o'clock, my friend and I put on the teakettle. We wanted to sit and chat before going to bed. Then we heard a creak as the old woman's bedroom door opened. She came into the kitchen and insisted on reading to us from her book of daily contemplations. To my distress, I saw that before she got to the last page, she turned back three pages. Over and over, she read those same three pages. Perhaps she was afraid of being alone in the dark or was feeling the approach of death.

Although frustrated, I kept a lid on my emotions. I stood there thinking, "Why doesn't she let go? I'm the helper, and she's the old woman. She should let me go to bed. Isn't it natural that I should feel bored and exhausted? I need a break. She's the one who has to give in." I was determined to hold on to my victimhood and anger.

What contrariness paralyzed me? As I thought about it later, I wondered if I had been trying to hang on to my view of myself as a super caregiver. Blaming her, I forgot to look at my own self-deception. My energy was stuck in controlling, frozen irritation. Could I have let go of my hesitation and suggested that we listen to the rest of the book tomorrow? At the very least, I might have suggested that we sit down and read in the living room. Was this old woman, who probably could feel what I was hiding from myself, trying to force me to get more real?

Relax your panic. It is easy to feel that you are alone in the world with no resources. It is as if you create an energetic shield around yourself. You lose your sense of being. You stop feeling connected to others and become an isolated bundle of worry. How can you relax when there is so much to worry about? You get so tight with anxiety, you become shielded from the help that you need.

I was often paralyzed by ideas about how my own father's care should go. My father had been living with my sister Judy for a year. At one point he was in the hospital for many months, trying to get over a staph infection that he had picked up in the hospital. He was determined to get well. He raged at the doctors for not helping him enough. When he was home with Judy, he raged at her, declaring, "I don't want to live here."

Although my family was scattered, we saw ourselves as a closed unit. We didn't know how to open our world and get some outside help. I alternated with my other sister, traveling from Vermont to California to try to help. In California I worried about my son, who was attending high school in Vermont. My sisters and I all had different ideas about how to proceed. Intense feelings often arise among family members over the care of a parent. Although I had seen it in others for years, I was surprised to find the same intensity in myself. I think my panic was increased by the thought that I, a professional caregiver, should know what to do.

Then I remembered. *Relax your panic.* Forget about what you do and don't know, what you should or should not do, and give yourself a chance to just be. I use meditation and contemplative exercises to help increase my sense of being. Another method is to simply sit with the worry as it escalates, waiting until it loses its momentum. Insight comes in the space that follows the worry, if you don't get stuck in your own habitual responses.

When I relaxed my worry about my father, events sorted themselves out to everyone's benefit. I realized I had been thinking of him as the same person he had been when I was a child. I began to see him as a human being and to think about his strengths instead of dwelling on his problems. I listened to all the people in his world: his wife, my sisters, friends, doctors, and the minister from the church. I saw that late in life he had fallen deeply in love with his second wife. Love had become more important than business. Even with all of the problems, there was a richness and strength in his relationship with Eleanor. His care evolved from the strength of that marriage. Caring for my father became a continual process of opening and giving in to the realities of his wishes and needs, to the reality of the family's needs, and to resources within the community.

Look for little gaps of openness. What might initially appear to be confusion in the elder may, in fact, be the beginning of more openness. Many people who have always been stubborn and determined begin to lighten their resolve in old age. Little gaps of openness allow caregivers the opportunity to bring attention to the spirit of the moment. But we have to be alert and intuitive to catch these moments.

Carla is a caregiver who is good at using her intuition. She once worked with an old woman who was so restless and confused that Carla had to drive her around, sometimes five times a day. Carla was getting a little burned out from so much driving. One day, as the old woman got up and headed for the door for the umpteenth time, Carla thought to herself, "Oh, no, here we go again." She walked the elder out to the car. It was early evening. As they reached the gate, the woman hesitated ever so slightly. She had forgotten why she was there. Carla saw an opportunity in the hesitation. She said, "Would you like to go inside and watch a movie? We have a good film." The old woman agreed.

In a flash, Carla saw that the elder was trying to relieve her anxiety in the only way she knew how—by going for a drive. Instead of doing what she would habitually do, Carla had recognized the opportunity to step into the gap in the forward momentum. It was a kind of magic. Instead of driving around for an hour over the same old roads, they sipped a glass of sherry and enjoyed a film.

In our society, where we know too much and feel too little, it takes practice to work creatively. Caregivers often try too hard, thinking that they have to listen to every word the elder says instead of feeling the atmosphere. Resentment and claustrophobia build, whereas acknowledgment and humor are needed.

John is a caregiver who is good at bringing in humor to create a light, warm environment. One day his client was asking over and over, "Where's Henry?" (Henry was her husband, who had died.) She asked the question fifty or a hundred times. John was standing at the refrigerator getting ready to prepare dinner when the old woman asked again, "Where's Henry?"

"Henry died, and we put him in the refrigerator," John answered. The old woman, looking startled, walked over to the refrigerator. As she put her hand on the door, she stopped and looked at John. "You're kidding, aren't you?" They both laughed, and the obsessive questioning stopped.

Caregivers can help elders let go of their own fear of enjoyment. Sharon kept repeating over and over, "Gerry has stolen my underwear." When Sharon started making accusations, her helper would take her out, maybe to a nearby restaurant. They would order hamburgers and salads, and Sharon would watch the people at nearby tables. "Do you see that woman with her hair dyed red?" Sharon would ask. Her state of mind switched from concern with herself to interest in others, a good first step toward widening the scope of a life.

When Susan served her client a glass of juice, the old woman picked it up and threw it on the sofa, barely missing her dog. Then she picked up her glass of water and threw that on the sofa, too. Susan said, "Maybe we could get your dog to move over so he could have a bath." The elder didn't laugh, but the tension was broken, and she refrained from throwing any more beverages.

Caregivers can use difficult situations as opportunities to introduce into the elder's life a moment of surprise that prepares the ground for the elder's letting go.

TIPS FOR EMBRACING THE ELDER'S WORLD

Slow down before you enter the elder's world. Put your hand on the doorknob, feel the metal of the knob, and turn it slowly. Walk into the house; don't hurry. Notice any change in the atmosphere from the outside to the inside. Is the temperature different? What about the texture of the air—is it lighter outside and heavier inside, or vice versa? Slowly hang up your coat, put down your packages, drop the trappings of the speedy world that you have left behind. Then sit down. Notice your body on the chair. Feel your back and arms. Slowly begin to notice the elder and the environment. What is your state of mind? Can you determine the elder's state of mind?

Trust the profound bond that brought you together. Don't talk too much. Sit quietly, drink tea, share a meal. Listen to the silence as well as to the voice of the parent or elder in your care. Realize that the elder is your teacher, showing you the way to let go, to be old.

Acknowledge your own feelings when fulfilling the requests of others. If your father demands that you type his life story and make forty copies immediately, and you feel resentful, acknowledge the resentment. Let the resentment fill your body. Breathe in black, then switch and breathe out white. Breathe in hot and black, breathe out cool and white. Then, from that state of mind, take whatever action you must take. You can't change the dynamic of your father's need to demand. What you can do is to acknowledge your feelings, at least to yourself.

Pay attention to the desires of the old person. If an old man tells you he's decided to memorize a book and spend the rest of his life reciting it, silently acknowledge the feeling tone that surrounds the desire. Appreciate the gumption of the plan. Support the elder's spirit, by feeling both the complaint and the longing that surrounds it. Then, if you can, create the environment to help carry out the plan: a comfortable chair to sit in, perhaps a tape recorder, and a celebratory supper after a long day of reciting. Staying connected to our elders can lead us from sadness to celebration.

EXERCISE: *Dealing with Silence*

Often elders who are frail have let go of the need to talk. They don't give the helper much feedback. It's like taking care of the sky—it's just there. If you are feeling bewildered by a silent elder, try going outside and looking at the sky. Lie on the grass with your arms and legs spread wide or just sit in a chair and look up. Instead of trying to figure out the elder's state of mind, expand your own until it's like the sky. This will perk you up. Your well-being will then spread to the elder.

PART THREE

THE REALITIES

———◄o►———

Working with Difficult Behaviors

L ATE ONE SUMMER AFTERNOON, as I drove home from the grocery store, my beeper went off. One of the helpers was sick, so I went to spend the evening with Gladys. I didn't know her evening routine. As I entered her little stone house, I nervously dropped my keys and stubbed my toe. I slipped a little on the braided rug that she refused to let us move. I helped her with her slippers before she had put her nightgown on. That violation of her routine threw her into a frenzy. She waved her cane at me, shouting, "Out, cat, crow, armhole."

All I could do was stand still, letting her agitation flow through me, until we both settled down. Then I said, "How about some dinner?" Gladys sat at her dining room table next to a window, through which she could see her bird feeder and the gazebo with pink roses climbing up the trellis. I mixed up an omelet in the adjoining kitchen. The birds pecked at their evening meal. Big black crows sat on the trellis watching Gladys.

At supper she mixed her peas with her potatoes and made a mess. Then she settled down and ate. "Cats eat birds," she told me. Finally, I understood. "Out, cat, crow, armhole" was a kind of poem about the panic and fear that birds and old ladies share.

One of the most disturbing and difficult situations that a caregiver has to confront is an elder who is confused, disoriented, and perhaps hostile. This chapter explains how these and other patterns of behavior develop and how—even if you can't solve the problem—you can learn to avoid the stagnation that can result and bring fresh energy to the situation.

There are several basic behavior patterns that old people often display as they slip from lives of doing into lives of being. A great many elders suffer from increasing memory loss. Some experience restlessness and want to wander about. Some are angry or combative. Some want to dominate others, either directly or indirectly. Some, especially if they are highly intelligent and perceptive, become overly critical. Some get caught in patterns of ignoring or denial. If the elder is also very stubborn, conflicts can become heated. She may be overly demanding or manipulative, playing one person off against another.

Old age lays bare our most basic needs. A person with a clear and penetrating mind might have learned that it isn't skillful to criticize others. But in old age, loss of memory might have dissolved his social conditioning, causing him to blurt out his observations with no regard for whether they sound polite. A person who was possessive of her mate might have learned to fill her days with activities. But in old age, with the loss of those activities, she might feel abandoned when she is left alone. Clinging behavior is accentuated when there is memory loss. The caregiver might simply have gone into the kitchen to cook, but the elder forgets that and feels all alone.

It isn't easy to keep a clear mind when someone is acting out. The temptation when working with a difficult elder is to let yourself get drawn into a neurotic state of mind so that you feel agitated or depressed. If you are working with a particularly difficult person, especially if that person is your parent, you will have to go beyond creating care plans and enriching the elder's world. You will have to work together with others to gently but firmly surround your parent with loving-kindness. The general approach is to look at the difficult behavior, then create a circle of support that enfolds conflict—effectively reinforcing the elder's strengths while learning to work with your own negative responses to his or her neurotic behavior. You support the elder's sanity so that the obstacles to positive expression can fall away. At the same time, you work on calming your panic, cutting through your own obstacles, and gaining greater clarity of mind.

Begin by asking yourself these questions: Do I need help? Do I need to bring more formality, stronger boundaries, and more discipline into the elder's life? Into my own life? Can I resolve this difficulty? Can I learn to live with the fact that there is no way to resolve it? Having accepted the situation, how can I make it as good as it can be? Don't worry about finding answers for the moment. Just use the questions as a way of relaxing and putting yourself in a more receptive frame of mind before proceeding.

We'll begin by examining these patterns of behavior in more detail.

CONFUSION

Confusion often results from a combination of several factors. First, there might be some physical problem: one or more strokes, Alzheimer's, or some other serious illness or condition. It could be simple exhaustion, the cumulative effect of one or more medications, or even the approach of death.

Even an elder who suffers from none of these things can have ample reason for confusion. You know the feeling of walking outside on a hot summer day. Instead of letting the heat penetrate you, you resist it. "Yuck. It's too hot. I shouldn't have to suffer like this." You confirm your image of yourself to ward off the direct experience of the heat. Resisting the heat, you begin to feel like a victim of the sun.

Now imagine that degree of physical difficulty, your resistance to it, and the barriers you erect to protect you from the experience multiplied tenfold. Can you see how such difficulty and resistance might lead to confusion? A constant attitude of complaint disconnects us from our experience, makes us feel like victims, and leads to a perpetual sense of burden. It isolates us from the rich possibilities that life presents. And eventually it leads into the deluded state of confusion.

The second factor in confusion is psychological—a feeling of uncertainty and fear. When people feel pain and fear, the tendency is to panic and try to control it. The more they try to control it, the more confused they become.

When you are with someone who suffers from confusion, you are always working at two levels. You are working with the person's basic being, which is expressed through longing—for his past life, for all the things he has lost, for feelings of groundedness and connection; and you are working with his fear—fear of his unconnected present and uncertain future. A person might forget his image of himself, might forget faces and words, might lose his social conditioning, but he doesn't forget his habitual responses to fear.

Finally, confusion may have a sociological component as well. Both elders and those who care for them sometimes take on society's view that since a person is old, she must be senile. In some cultures, when an elder appears to be confused, the family and community trust that the elder is opening up and communing with the gods. In this way, the spirit of old age is respected, and there is a community structure to accommodate the divergent behavior.

In our culture, with dispersed families and weakened communities, eccentricity is not so easy to accommodate. It tends to be labeled as an illness. Medications and social services are brought to bear, in an attempt to reduce the confusion or dull it. Then the old people who are labeled and judged lose trust in themselves, and their state of mind declines according to society's expectations.

Many elders are acting out patterns of confusion in response to a cultural environment in which feelings are not recognized. For instance, an elder might understandably feel sad because of the loss of a loved one or because her life didn't turn out the way she wanted. If that sadness is labeled as depression, the elder might blame herself for falling into low spirits, and her self-esteem erodes. If the spirit of old age is not respected and encouraged, patterns of confusion solidify.

When Edith, who had had a series of small strokes, found out that her caregiver, Marjorie, was leaving to go to graduate school, she accused her of stealing. I visited Edith to find out more about it. "What has been stolen?" I asked. "A cookie and a dish towel," she said. Even as Edith heard her own words, she realized that she was making it up. Who would want to steal a cookie and a dish towel?

Yet Edith knew that *something* had been stolen; when Marjorie left, she would miss her. She covered up her fear of emptiness by making accusations. She went from accusing Marjorie to accusing herself of having made a mistake. "Forgive me, I'm a senile old lady," she said. The next day Edith climbed up on a little stool, fell off, and hurt her back. For several days, she lay on her sofa repeating over and over, "Pride goeth before a fall. Pride goeth before a fall."

The confusion of isolation often develops this way. Edith feared the feeling of emptiness, so she fell back upon self-blame. Her tool of control was repetition of a statement: "Pride goeth before a fall." Edith was obsessed. She wanted everyone to know that she had made a mistake and that she knew the cause. She was isolating herself with her pride. She controlled with repetition. The more she blamed herself, the more mistakes she made. Her energy was stuck.

Edith had certain qualities that helped her overcome her isolation and confusion. She was willing to expose her confusion to others. She wanted to communicate and to teach her helpers the dangers of pride. And she was fortunate to have a good circle of support. Her helpers didn't believe that because she was old, she had to be senile. Their task was to see her pride as a smoke screen that covered the spirit of her being and to surround her obstacle with warmth, humor, and insight. The caregivers were relaxed enough to figure out what to do. They called Edith's hero, the minister from her church, who came to see her. "Edith, you need to develop more humility," he told her with a smile. Edith laughed. For a time, she was no longer confused. Edith's willingness to reveal and the circle's willingness to accept had worked together to create an environment in which Edith could gradually relax.

Memory Loss

Many people past the age of fifty experience some loss of memory. Memory is not a tangible organ like the brain. It is a part of our existence that we construct over the years by filtering experience in such a way as to build a seemingly solid image of ourselves. Memory is convenient and reassuring, but it is possible to have a normal life with very little long-term memory.

Memory loss becomes more difficult when someone can't remember what happened five minutes ago. The loss of short-term memory leads to several distressing symptoms. A person might lose much of his sense of self, but the basic, bare-bones ego remains, with its complaints, restlessness, anxiety, and depression. His inner discipline might remain as well, and a feeling of longing. Whatever is left is what you have to work with.

The loss of memory per se is not the problem. What creates confusion is disconnection. When loss of memory disconnects a person from outer relationships and from trust in her inner strength, then difficulties arise. Disconnections might show themselves in peculiar ways. One day I was with an old woman who was wringing her hands and crying. "My hands are cold," she said. But in fact, her feet had gotten wet where snow had seeped into her boots. Dry socks took care of her cold hands. Somehow this woman had lost the connection between what she felt and what she thought. Mind and body were not working together.

On another occasion, I had spent a relaxed and enjoyable evening with an old woman whose mind and body seemed to be in harmony. As I prepared to help her into bed, she asked me, "Did you put down the anchor?" She thought we were on a boat. Her body was working, but her location was off.

It is difficult to go forward with life when memory of the past is gone and prospects for the future are dim. Some people become so disconnected from any sense of direction that they don't know whether they should go this way or that. I used to drive a woman who would always tell me, "We're going the wrong way." If we were driving north, she thought we should go south. If we were driving south, she insisted on going north.

With no sense of direction, an elder might fall into despair, as the future stretches out long and gray. When people become disconnected from reference points such as work and hopes for the future, they lose their sense of self. Without memory of who they are, what distinction, emotional or physical, can they feel between themselves and others? One old woman was traveling on the freeway with her two daughters when a large truck whizzed by. "Are we a truck?" she asked.

Many old people go over and over past events, trying to maintain their sense of themselves. "I went to camp when I was five," an old woman used to tell me again and again. Some people repeat stories. Others ask the same questions time after time: "When are we going?" "What day is it?" Often it seems to be an attempt to fill the empty space left by weak memory. Caring for someone with short-term memory loss can be as wearing as listening to a leaky faucet at midnight.

Loss of short-term memory may also lead to a sense of extreme loneliness, as if the person had lost a best friend. Someone without memory may try to cling to family or to a caregiver and may be unable to tolerate being left alone for long. Sharon could remember only a few highlights from the past. She spent hours straightening her shelves and drawers. Like many people who suffer from short-term memory loss, she developed rigid routines and repetitions, which provided some security and alleviated her fear of being alone.

Suspicions develop easily for someone without memory. A woman once asked me, as we pulled out into traffic, if the car windows were bulletproof. Many elders suspect that no one cares. Who can trust relationships or the environment when a visit is forgotten five minutes after the visitor leaves?

Losing track of one's location in time and space is also common with memory loss. One elderly woman, returning from a family gathering, told her helper how nice it had been to see her grandmother at the reunion. Her grandmother, of course, had been dead for many years. Elders often seem to see people from their past in the present moment. It is as if the grid of past, present, and future that helps a person organize his world has dissolved. This isn't usually a problem, as long as helpers don't make an issue of it.

Delusions develop easily when memory is weak. A delusion is a self-deception that a person insists is true. My father had lost his grasp on the past, so he tried to rewrite his future. He defined himself as a man who owned a business. Although he had many talents, he did not consider himself a worthwhile person unless he owned a business.

It would have been natural for my father to grieve the losses in his life. After all, he had lost his parents, his brothers, his first wife, his business, and his health. But his emotional life had not been nurtured; he thought he was supposed to be invincible, always cheerful. He covered over his feelings of failure by spending his days imagining ways to make money. He rewrote a happy ending to his story, which became a delusion, unshakably held, that he had won millions of dollars. Listening to him made me crazy with frustration, but I also could feel his longing, his spirit calling out for fulfillment. His imagined good luck was an expression of that spirit. I chose to respond to the generosity of his spirit instead of to his madness.

"What would you do with the money?" I asked. "I'll give a million to the church and a million to each of you girls," he answered. Then he relaxed, and we could talk about other things. Whenever I forgot to keep his longing in mind, trouble would arise. If I tried to argue with him—"No, you haven't won any money"—he would become furious, run to the phone, and try to call his accountant. When confused people are making a last stand with their bare-bones ego, opposition does not help; communication does.

RESTLESSNESS AND WANDERING

People who suffer from short-term memory loss, perhaps from damage to the brain, often experience restlessness as well. Sometimes it is the result of boredom, especially the boredom that comes with the loss of a sense of direction in life. People who feel abandoned often restlessly search for something they feel is missing. It is exhausting, both for themselves and for their caregivers.

Wandering is one of the most frightening behaviors that elders manifest, because of the danger of their getting hurt. Try to have a safe place where the person can wander unattended—a fenced yard or a secure room. Although no one should wander for long periods of time, sometimes if a person wanders for a while, it helps him to get in touch with his own energy, so he can relax and settle down. The challenge is to find something that draws him back.

Occasionally, a person wanders because there is not enough sense of direction for the day, just as the mind wanders when there is no focus. With the loss of memory, the elder may find it hard to recall what to do or what prospects the day holds, so a well-planned day helps. Write out a daily schedule of enjoyable events and go over it with the elder, as discussed in Chapter 5.

Don't be afraid to acknowledge the elder's confusion. One evening Ellen insisted on going out the door. It was dark, so she hesitated and said, "I have to get to the train." Her caregiver gently said, "You don't know where you are, do you?" Ellen startled as if she were waking up. She looked at her helper and said, "No, I don't." The helper then acknowledged how hard it is to feel confused. Ellen relaxed and went back into the house.

MOOD SWINGS AND HALLUCINATIONS

Serious mood swings afflict many elders. The caregiver should be prepared for unpredictable behavior. On one day, the person may be excitable, arrogant, aggressive, or restless; on another day, that same person may feel depressed, not want to eat, and be apologetic and humble.

When someone suffers from mood swings, it helps to maintain a rhythm of routine and discipline in the daily schedule. Depending on which part of the cycle a person is in, the emphasis should vary. On the low side of the cycle, more activity is needed. Socializing with a variety of people may help. When the elder has become overly excited, rest can be encouraged as well as staying in and eating good food.

In some cases, the excitement is so pronounced that caregivers have to go with the flow of the energy until it wears itself out. The elder may need to walk, go for a drive, or enter into the chaos of a large-group gathering, such as a fair, a crowded restaurant, or a busy shopping area. Whether the elder is low or high, the daily schedule should be followed as closely as possible.

Some old people, at the slightest hint of rejection, retreat from the "real" world into a hallucinatory world of dreams. Elizabeth filled her empty world with hallucinations of little children, who inhabited her house by day and sat on the back fence wailing at night. Dorothy, in the loneliness after her son committed suicide, also filled her world with little people. When I visited her house one day, I made the mistake of sitting on one of them. "Don't you see them?" she asked me. I had to tell her that I could not.

A doctor should be consulted when hallucinations occur. They can arise from a neurological disorder, exhaustion, or medication. Whatever their cause, hallucinations need to be respected and approached with an open mind. I have often suspected that the very frail have pierced through the veils that limit our earthbound vision and see what we cannot. Many fragile elders stand with their feet in two worlds—the physical world of aches and pains and the incorporeal world of spirit and dreams.

Recently an old woman got up in the middle of the night and called her helper. "Help me," she said, "the water is rising." She had rolled her pajama bottoms up to her knees and seemed to be wading in water. The caregiver took the old woman by the arm, led her out to the living room, wrapped her in a warm shawl, built a fire in the fireplace, and made her a cup of warm milk. They sat together, watching the fire and reading. The woman calmed down and went back to bed.

The next day another caregiver, who had not been working that night, called to tell me about a dream she had had in which this same old woman appeared and led her down into another world to find the family burial vaults. At the bottom of this other world, a big door opened out onto a black sea, rolling with waves. A sailboat floated on the sea, and the two women stepped into the boat and sailed away. As the caregiver told me her dream, I thought of the old woman wading in the imaginary water. For a moment I wondered, What is real and what is imaginary?

MISTRUST AND OVERCONTROLLING

A pattern of mistrust and overcontrolling is one of the most difficult situations to work with. Although many elderly people are mistrustful of a new caregiver in the beginning, sometimes the mistrust continues, and they won't allow anyone in. How can you provide needed care and safety for an elder who refuses help? The caregiver and the family have to support each other. The elder will try to drive the helper away and is likely to succeed unless the helper is patient and is backed by the family.

The movie *Driving Miss Daisy* is a good portrayal of this dilemma. The helper in the film is humble, patient, shrewd, and in need of a job. Miss Daisy doesn't want help and tries to drive him away by accusing him of theft and by keeping her distance. The film describes their gradually developing friendship over a period of years, against a backdrop of racial prejudice and evaporating family connections. It shows the kind of caring relationship that can develop in spite of demanding and mistrust, against all odds.

CRITICIZING AND DEMANDING

When an elder is overly critical or demanding, you may feel like covering up your hurt or striking back in anger. It isn't easy to absorb criticism without taking it personally and without responding with aggression, especially when the elder is your parent. But remember that a person who is critical of others is usually equally hard on himself.

Sometimes provocative remarks are a way (albeit a negative one) of trying to get attention. Fighting and criticizing are sometimes attempts to express intimacy. Whatever the trigger for the negativity, acknowledge your own feelings, but don't act them out. The material in Chapter 6 on enriching the elder's state of mind might help here.

Little flashes of insight often come just when we think we are stuck in some impossible situation. Helen was a difficult woman to care for. Every day she would call my office and complain that Barbara, her helper, had stolen her silver candlesticks. Each morning when Helen made her accusation, I would defend the helper. "No, Helen, Barbara didn't steal them. You gave them to her for her wedding shower." "That's a lie," Helen would respond. "She stole them, and I'm calling the police." We would go back and forth like that until one or the other of us hung up. One day, as she threatened to call the police, I had a little flash of insight. I realized that complaining was her way of communicating. Instead of defending Barbara or myself, I thanked Helen warmly for advising me of her concerns. "Helen, I really appreciate your letting me know about this," I said. "Well, I thought you would want to know," she answered. We went on to have a friendly conversation, and she never mentioned the candlesticks again.

COMBATIVE BEHAVIOR

When a person loses his sense of himself, he may become excessively willful. This willfulness may lead to explosive, even combative, behavior. It can take the form of not wanting to change clothes or refusing to bathe. He feels his existence is threatened, so he fears any kind of change.

It isn't always clear what causes a frail old person to suddenly become violently angry. Sometimes it is frustration at not being able to perform some function. Maybe the elder has been approached too abruptly; it is good to signal the transition from one activity to another: "Now that you're dressed, shall we walk out to the living room?"

As soon as the distress settles, approach the elder gently with some expression of warm physical presence. Fran once threw a glass of cranberry juice at a guest, then got up to walk out the door. The guest got Fran's coat and helped her with it, put a scarf around her neck, and smoothed it out. He put his arm around her and gave her a hug. As I watched, I could see the tension leave Fran's body.

Nearly all instances of combative behavior can be solved with a strong supportive presence. Most aggression is brief. When it's over, it helps to go right back to the regular routine, as if nothing had happened. If everyone in a circle of care is feeling angry or territorial, it may be a signal that some kind of manipulation is coming from the center of the circle. Some old people (as well as some helpers) like to play one person off against another. Manipulation only works, however, if the person being manipulated agrees to it.

WORKING WITH DIFFICULT BEHAVIOR

Working with difficult behavior patterns is an ongoing process. There's no quick and easy solution. Here are a number of approaches that can help to lighten the situation, even if they can't make the behavior go away:

Examine your own state of mind. Do you feel frightened or worried about how to respond? Are you afraid that you won't be able to calm the elder down? Are you afraid you will be up all night? Have you fallen into your own bare-bones ego, thinking, "I'm supposed to be a helper, but I feel like a victim instead"?

Be fearless about acknowledging your true feelings. Notice ways in which you struggle against yourself. For instance, notice whether you blame yourself for your parent's confusion. Notice whether you feel guilty that you are out working instead of taking care of your parent. You may be blaming yourself for responding to larger social forces over which you have little control. Notice whether you keep thinking, "This isn't the way it should be."

Don't worry about what might be required in the future. Concentrate on the here and now. Instead of thinking about what should happen, notice what is happening, without judging or trying to change it. Look at where the energy is stuck and at any longing that surrounds it. Acknowledge the discomfort of feeling stuck. Just noticing and acknowledging the feeling of a situation releases energy. Let yourself appreciate what is occurring. It is an opportunity for learning, an opportunity to develop more compassion.

Breathe in tension, breathe out calm. If you feel that the confusion of an older person is stirring your anxiety, intensify your tension for a moment. Imagine taking into yourself, with your breath, your own and the elder's discomfort as well as the discomfort of all people who are feeling stuck. Don't try to figure out to whom the panic belongs or where it came from. Just let the chaos tighten your body for a moment, as if you were a lightning rod for panic. Let the discomfort fill your body, your mind, the room. Welcome it; heighten it.

Then breathe out, purposely sending out a feeling of humor and lightness and well-being. Ground the panic by engaging in some simple activity. Make a cup of tea and focus all of your attention on the process of brewing, serving, and drinking the tea, then washing out the teapot.

If you calm yourself, the elder's anxiety will diminish for a while. The intention to take upon yourself the suffering of another and to give back well-being is often enough to shift the energy of the situation. When the calming occurs, relax and do something enjoyable with the elder. Go out for lunch together, play a game of cards or Scrabble, go for a walk or a drive. Restore your sense that life holds many joys and pleasures.

This practice also works with resentment. If you are feeling resentful because of something the old person said to you, or resentful that you have too much to do, acknowledge the way you are feeling. Heighten the resentment by breathing it in, until it fills your whole body. Then let go. On the out breath, breathe out a feeling of peace, healthiness, and well-being.

Often caregivers are able to do the first part of this practice. They can take on the suffering of the old or the resentment, but then they forget to complete the exchange, to drop the resentment and let the peace emerge. A hospice nurse once told me, "Be like a sponge: absorb the negativity, but don't forget to squeeze out the sponge and start fresh."

One of the most useful but difficult practices is to do nothing: just wait, listen, without jumping to conclusions. If you try to do too much, what you do might be more harmful than helpful. You might sink into the old person's depression. You might try to avoid your own life by sacrificing yourself to the needs of the elder. You might find yourself trying to please the elder just to keep her quiet. You might become too tight and rigid, then burst out in a rage. It often takes a long while before situations are revealed to the point of clarity. In the meantime, it is perfectly all right to sit quietly and feel the depth of your exhaustion and resentment. Eventually a little spark of something bright and new will reignite your life force. Then you begin to notice your surroundings: the big belly of a pregnant hospice nurse, purple irises in a glass vase, the acrid smell of bleach on the bedpan. That is the beginning of noticing how to take care of yourself and others.

Attend to the elder's physical condition. Whenever unusual or difficult behavior appears in an elderly person, it is important that he have a physical examination by a good doctor. High blood pressure, vitamin deficiencies, metabolic disorders, hydrocephalus, strokes, chronic infections of brain tissue, and high blood cholesterol levels are some of the conditions that can contribute to behavioral changes, as can depression, exhaustion, poor nutrition, and the cumulative effects of medication. An elder who has been in the hospital for an extended stay may become temporarily confused as a result of stimulus deprivation.

But even if the elder is diagnosed with a physical condition, don't attach too much importance to the label. Instead, look at the whole pattern: look at the person's being as well as the symptomatic behavior. Family members and caregivers who are working with difficult situations would often give anything to have a pill that would help the person's state of mind. But it's hard to find pills that work well over a long period of time. An antipsychotic drug might be given to an elder who is revved up or overanxious. The pill might be valuable in the short run, but if it is given over an extended period, the same medicine might lead to rigidity of limbs and rigidity of behavior. When my father was in a manic state, a medicine helped to calm him down. But over time it made him so rigid that he would sit for hours looking at his watch to see if it was time for his wife, Eleanor, to come. Once the medication had done its work, it needed to be discontinued.

Medication should be seen as simply one factor in the whole plan of care. Antianxiety pills might help an elder, but only if used as part of a complete understanding of the anxious state of mind. The circle of care must work to cheer up the environment around the anxiety. Likewise with antidepressants. Is the medicine treating a real depression, or is it an attempt to perk up the low spirits of an elder in order to make the caregiver feel better?

The most important point about medications is to find a doctor who understands the unique needs of the elderly. The doctors who have impressed me most have been conservative about medications, have used them as a last resort, have gradually reduced dosages after the medications have worked, have prescribed smaller doses for frail systems, and have monitored dosages carefully for side effects or for damage to liver or kidneys.

Don't be afraid to consult a doctor about medications to help with confusional disorders. But don't think that a pill will solve your problems. If you do use medication, use it as part of a more comprehensive effort to address the confusion. Nurses, social workers, gerontologists, and other experts in your community can give you practical tips about what might help.

Attend to the elder's basic being. If you are a caregiver to someone old, there often isn't much you can do either to remedy the person's physical condition or to talk her out of her views. What you can do is address what I call the "bare-bones ego." I remember the first time I heard the term. My former partner, Vicky Howard, and I had just returned from visiting one of our clients, Pearl. No matter what Vicky or I said to this frail little woman, she responded the same way: "My knees hurt. My eyes don't work. Richard Nixon let us down." Afterward Vicky looked at me and said, "Now there's a case of bare-bones ego." I thought to myself, "That's it— Pearl's energy is stuck in an unending loop; she's reduced to her bare-bones ego."

Pearl, like many elders, had lost a great deal in her eighty-eight years— her husband, her work, her health, and her faculties. Like many others who have lost the precious attachments of their lives, she complained. But she had gone beyond saying, "I am Pearl, and this shouldn't be happening to me." Her loss had intensified to the point of taking away even her basic sense of herself.

Her complaint was more bare-bones. It was a smoke screen to cover her fear of the loss of herself. She couldn't directly grieve for herself, but she knew she felt uncomfortable. She complained about her eyes and about politics. It was the last stand of ego, the last resistance to the pain of her genuine loss.

There was some kind of blockage between Pearl's head and her heart. That blockage was her bare-bones ego. With the flow of her energy blocked, she felt stuck. She felt separate, isolated from herself and her world. In her loneliness, it almost seemed that her complaint had become her entertainment and comfort. It filled the emptiness of her days. But there was longing, too. She didn't want to complain just to herself. She wanted at least to tell someone else about her troubles. It is this longing for connection that provides a way out of confusion.

Many elders live in a world that is small and full of frustration. Life seems to spiral downward and inward until the atmosphere becomes closed in and claustrophobic. Some old people who find themselves isolated in this way may attempt to hide their isolation. Others try in various ways to burst out of it.

An old woman sat in the living room of the house where she had lived for forty years. She was surrounded by evidence of a full, rich life—paintings, books, family pictures, the precious objects gathered over ninety years of living. Suddenly she said to me, "Won't you take me home? I want to go home." She stood up on wobbly legs and headed for the door.

The day had been a pleasant one of nice meals, reading and listening to music, and a visit from a friend for tea. But by five o'clock, nothing seemed familiar to this old woman. Did some circulation to the brain diminish? Was it in the transition from afternoon to evening that a sense of loneliness crept up on her? Why had she disconnected from the comforts of the day?

Even in good health it's not always easy to stay connected to the present moment. In old age, the ecology of body and mind is more delicate. Something as simple as losing your keys can throw you out of balance. You can't find your keys, you wonder if you're losing your memory, then you panic and close a drawer on your finger.

With the approach of evening, this elder fell back on her bare-bones ego: "I am a woman abandoned. This isn't my home." What she was saying was, "I feel uncomfortable because the day has ended and the night has not yet begun. Transitions are difficult for me. I feel lost. I want to feel better."

Look to see where the elder's world has narrowed. Is she repeating herself? Is he sitting in a chair all day doing nothing? Is she stuck in agitation or delusion? Ask yourself how you can bring some fresh air into her narrowed world. What is her fear of stepping out? What is her fear of staying in? Look at ways to get the energy circulating around the confusion. Remember, all of us long for love and connection, and all of us resist it. All of us fall into confusion, but confusion can relax. The task is to recognize the bare-bones ego, then surround it with warmth, humor, and respect.

One thing you can do in working with confused people is to intervene in their isolation. Confusion and isolation feed on each other. Isolation leads to confusion; confusion, whether it comes from a tangled brain or a broken heart, further isolates a person from feeling the wholeness of existence. The first step is to identify the disconnection. How has the person become disconnected from her world? Can you help her become reconnected?

Remember that confusion is not who that elder is, merely what he's manifesting at the time. Nor is it necessarily permanent. It is a smoke screen that keeps people from experiencing their basic sense of being. Whether a person has a brain disorder or a psychological disorder, his basic being is not disturbed. What is disturbed is the ability to process what is received so that it can be communicated in a meaningful way. Caregiving is learning to stir and release the stagnation that can result from such obstacles.

Adjust the plan for the day. Without trying to change the elder's confusion, plan an event that the elder has enjoyed in the past. I remember one old woman who loved to play Scrabble. No matter how angry or confused she was, she would drop it to play a game of Scrabble. Another old woman who had lost the power of comprehensible speech was able to paint, with watercolors, scenes from happy times at the beach when she was a child.

A creative yet steady routine can help calm elders who are restless, moody, or disconnected. The most important point with restlessness, for example, is to appreciate the energy that a restless person has. People who suffer from boredom and restlessness are often highly intelligent. Appreciate that the elder may not have developed an inner discipline to calm her restlessness. What is needed is a daily care plan that provides plenty of opportunity for the person to burn off energy in constructive ways, so that it doesn't escalate into combativeness or aimless wandering.

The following care notes show how the activities of the whole day created a light atmosphere around an elder's dark mood and restlessness:

7:30 AM   Mary got up. The caregiver took her to the bathroom and helped her to bathe and dress. Then Mary ate breakfast.

8:15   Mary got up from her breakfast. Her lips were moving, but she didn't speak. The expression on her face was grumpy. She started walking to the front door. The caregiver got Mary's coat and helped her to the car. They drove to the grocery store to shop. The helper got Mary to push the grocery cart around the store. Mary kept asking, "Do we have any money?" The helper told her, "Yes, we have money. Do you want asparagus or broccoli?"

9:30   Mary's daughter took her mother to a neighbor's for tea.

10:30   Mary returned from tea. She wouldn't sit down. Instead, she headed for the front door. The helper got her coat, and they went for a drive. On their way back from the drive, they came to a dirt road, and the helper slowed down. "You're trying to annoy me," Mary said. "What do you mean?" the helper asked. "You're going too slow," Mary said. "I'm trying not to slide on the ice," the helper replied. "If you go too slow, we'll get towed away," Mary said. "No, I'm just trying to keep us safe," responded the helper. "Well, if that's true, I'm grateful," said Mary.

12:00 N   While the caregiver prepared lunch, Mary sat quietly. As they ate lunch, Mary looked at her helper and asked, "Do you curl your hair?" The helper answered, "Yes, I get a permanent." "Well, you need another one," Mary said. It seemed as if she was trying to stir up some kind of trouble, but the caregiver took it in stride and agreed with Mary, saying, "Maybe you're right."

12:45 PM   Mary took a nap.

1:45 Mary got up from her nap. The caregiver built a fire, put on music, and served tea and cookies. A visitor came. Mary wouldn't drink her tea. She had it in mind that her visitor was going to take her for a drive. Mary kept saying, "Aren't we going?" Finally, the visitor and the caregiver took Mary for a drive, but Mary couldn't shed her dark spirits. She criticized the helper, her friend, even the weather.

3:30 Mary rested. After a while, she got up restless and bored. She wanted to go for another drive, but the caregiver got her to take a walk instead.

4:30 The caregiver got Mary to help with supper preparation. As Mary cut the asparagus and made a tray of cheese and crackers, her spirits lifted. She walked around her living room pointing out different objects and telling where she got them. She pointed to a Latin acronym carved on an old chest. "It means 'In this sign,'" she said. (The acronym, "IHS," is short for *In hoc signo vinces*, "In this sign [the Cross], you shall conquer.") She walked around chanting "In this sign." She said it over and over, and it seemed to build a celebratory mood. The helper joined the chanting. Finally, they sat on the sofa. Mary drank a glass of apple cider. She relaxed, watched the fire, then picked up a book and began to read.

6:30 Mary's daughter came for dinner. They ate and chatted.

8:00 Mary went to bed in a happy mood and slept through the night.

Mary's day started out bleak, but her restlessness and critical behavior were channeled into ordinary activity—shopping, seeing her daughter, visiting a friend, exercising, and riding in the car. The day had a rhythm of morning routines, afternoon routines, and evening routines, so Mary had a sense of forward movement through her day, which ended in a mood of celebration.

If the elder is unable to participate in domestic activity, explore the possibility of setting a time for reading to her or drawing with her, or instigate some type of physical activity. It helps to mark the boundary of the periods of the day, so that it doesn't just drift from one soap opera to the next. But even if the elder likes to watch television, make sure that the viewing is part of a disciplined schedule.

Mary had twenty-four-hour care, in which family, friends, neighbors, and helpers worked together. But even if a helper comes for only a few hours a day, she can be instructed in how to work with a daily schedule to help an elder release restless energy and create moments of celebration.

Slogans to Help You Work with Difficulty

Slogan practice can help you go beyond your discomfort into greater awareness. Slogans can be used to remind yourself of the wisdom inherent in every situation. Contemplate the meaning of the slogans at your leisure. Then, when a situation arises, the appropriate slogan will come to mind, and you can apply its wisdom. You can't keep two things in your mind at once. If something crazy happens, remembering a slogan can help transform the craziness with sanity. In that way, distress itself will provide the opening for sanity.

See all situations as passing memory. This slogan will help to release you from the pain of feeling burdened. Contemplate it while walking, while sitting in meditation, or when you're driving.

Sometimes when I'm writing and I get stuck, I go sit on my back porch. My yard is surrounded by very old trees, which I think of as warriors and protectors—tall and deep-rooted. My petty concerns seem so small next to the majesty of the trees. It is the same when I am with an elder who is expressing some resistance. I see that the present, irritating as it may be, is as transitory as a clock tick. In a moment too fleeting to measure, it will be memory. Sometimes this feeling brings sadness, but it can also bring lightness and playfulness.

I used to drive an old woman who kept repeating herself. As we drove along a highway next to a river, she would ask, "What is the name of that river?"

"That's the Passumpsic River," I would answer, and then she would ask again, over and over. For a moment, the day would stretch out, and I would feel enclosed in a small car driving down a road with an elder who repeatedly asked the same question. For a moment, I would think, "I can't stand this another minute." And then I would think how all situations are passing memory, and the feeling of burden would lighten. "That is the Passumpsic River," I would say, and then I would wonder, Is the river the water or the banks or the reflections of the clouds in the turbulent foam? "What is the name of that river?" she asked yet again. We had driven far south by this time. I looked out the car window and saw the river widening and realized that it had changed.

"That's the Connecticut River," I answered.

"Oh," she said. "I thought it was the Passumpsic." We turned around and went home, and she didn't ask that question again.

Notice everything; respect everything. This motto can revolutionize a caregiving relationship, shifting the balance from suspicion to trust. It also makes potentially dull work interesting. Most of us are in a hurry when we approach someone old. In our rush, we don't see with much precision.

When I would visit my father, before I had even sat down, I would tell him that I couldn't stay long. I was defending myself against some demand that I expected he would make. If the slogan came to mind, I would slow down. I would notice that he was sitting there waiting to see me and that he wanted something. I would notice that I felt resistance to the antici-pated demand and that it made me nervous.

I could respect the dynamic of what was taking place between us. He would ask me to phone a friend of his to request a favor. I didn't want to do it, but I hated to tell him no. When I got in touch with the dynamic of our interaction, I began to respect his right to make the request as well as my right to refuse. I was able to tell him that I was too shy to make the phone call. Communication opened between us.

Be steady; don't go up and down. Old people often have good days and terrible days. It is helpful if you don't rise and fall with the uncertainties of the day. On cheerful days, you can be lightly cheerful without going overboard into elation. On dark days, you can be lightly cheerful without sinking into depression.

If an old woman takes my hand and looks me in the eye and tells me that she wants to go home with me, I can experience her charm, and I can refuse to do what she wants. I can stay steady. Likewise, if she tells me I am an evil witch, I don't have to take it personally.

GIVING YOURSELF A BREAK

When you are caring for someone who is difficult, you often get up in the morning and ask yourself, "How can I get through another day?" Elders, especially our mothers and fathers, can sometimes push us over the edge, into a state of mind that is pretty uncomfortable. If you are feeling burned out, ask yourself whether you've taken on too much. Have you created a circle of care, or are you trying to do it all yourself? Are you afraid to trust others to help? Are you trying to please someone else at the expense of your own life? Are you approaching care as a path of mindfulness, wisdom, and appreciation, or are you using care as a way to be hard on yourself? Is your state of mind resentful or calm?

A lot of burnout has to do with unfulfilled expectations. We become attached to a self-image of sacrifice or accomplishment, thinking, "Look at me. I've sacrificed more than anyone. I'm a good person." We might fan the flame of resentment if we feel underappreciated. Caregivers are sensitive and idealistic people. If you've built your life around other people's approval, a life of fulfilling other people's needs and wants, eventually you will burn out. The helpers who tend to burn out are the ones who try to make caring a cause, a reason for being.

Watch for signs of imbalance in your own life. I remember once cleaning out an old man's car until it shone. When I got into my own car, I noticed that it was filled with unopened mail, overdue library books, and snow boots that had been in the backseat since the previous winter. The contrast between the old man's car and mine made me wonder if I had become overinvolved in his care. Overattention to his needs had become a way to avoid attending to my own life.

There are ways to turn the difficulty into an opportunity to develop more compassion, to make friends with yourself, to learn to see what is needed and trust it. Here are some suggestions:

Be truly present. If a parent or client is repeating himself, take a friend or relative with you for a visit. Spend fifteen minutes listening to the elder. Then switch; let your friend listen for fifteen minutes. Keep switching back and forth. While you are listening, pay close attention to what the person is saying. Pay attention to how he is dressed. Notice the room, the general atmosphere. When you are not on listening duty, leave the room. Go into the kitchen and make tea, or go outside. When you are on, be on. When you are off, be off.

Try a change of location. If you are with an elder who is agitated, confused, or repeating herself, don't try to change the confusion or calm it down. Instead, switch the location. If your mother is sitting on the sofa repeating herself, ask her if she would like to go for a drive or ask her to come sit at the kitchen table.

Savor the joy of simple connection. Sit with a confused elder. Listen to what he tells you and appreciate the communication. Don't worry about whether it is right or wrong, crazy or sane. Instead, enjoy the spirit of sharing. If you're with an elder who is sad and depressed, don't try to cheer him up; just be with the sadness. Is it his or yours? Does it matter? Can you be with it without trying to change it?

When I went to visit Vanessa, I found her lying in bed. Venetian blinds shut out the light of day. I helped her out of bed and into her robe. We walked into her sitting room. "This old age is a punishment for my whole life," she confided to me. Vanessa didn't pretend to feel good, and I didn't pretend that she should. For a moment, there were no pretenses or secrets. Then she pointed to a copper plate on the wall and began to tell me about her trip to Egypt.

That unguarded moment with Vanessa was like a cool drink on a hot summer day—real and refreshing. Too often we are so busy trying to make things right that we miss such refreshing moments altogether.

Try listening more than talking. Listen to the elder, to other family members, to doctors, nurses, and social workers. Acknowledge and take to heart what people tell you. This kind of communication will help you learn to circulate the energy around the confusion. Like the heart pumping blood and sending oxygen to the cells, the circulation of energy spreads ideas, messages. Confusion is a signal that the messages are not getting through. As a caregiver, you can find new pathways so communication can continue.

Ground yourself in memories of love and happiness. Spend five minutes at the beginning of each day remembering that your parents gave you life. Remember the way you loved your parents when you were a child. As you go through your day, extend that attitude to everyone you meet. Remember that all people want love and happiness.

CARE STUDY

Criticism and Caring

————◄○►————

Lane was a widow who dressed in black pants and big, blue denim shirts. At one time, she had been tall and good-looking; now she had shrunk to five feet and weighed seventy-five pounds. Two long tubes attached her to a tall, green oxygen tank, which fueled her breath of life.

Lane drank a manhattan for lunch and scotch at five. Sociability had been her life, but her love of a good time was tempered by a strict New England upbringing, which had taught her to work hard, save money, and fuss. "Don't sit on that chair," she would tell a visiting family member. Her concern for the fragile chair outweighed her appreciation of the family visit.

Lane worried about running out of lightbulbs, running out of cherries for the manhattans, and running out of breath. "What if the pipes freeze? What if I use up all my money?" She battled an unseen army of dirt, bugs, and helpers.

Lane posed an interesting dilemma for her caregivers. How could we take care of her without being sucked into her worry? How could we help her connect to her strength, which was her genuine interest in others? We had to acknowledge her fear without becoming fearful ourselves.

Lane's gift and her obstacle were often one and the same. She had a talent for making friends, but then she did not want to let them go. It was as if she trapped her friends in a web, torturing them with her complaints. She became despondent when they tried to leave. Any change in her environment—a friend's departure, running out of maraschino cherries, or losing her breath—sparked fear, which made her critical, emotional, and anxious.

Lane's worries ceased at 5:00 PM, when the house was as clean as one helper could get it that day and her papers were sorted into little piles with rubber bands around them. It was too late to weed and too early for dinner. Then Lane, reeling out the long cords that attached her to her oxygen tank, sat on her front porch to watch hummingbirds and to hold court. Friends and family gathered, while Lane wove a convivial web of sociability: drinks, snacks, and gossip. On some days, when Lane was well enough and the scotch had worked its magic, the friends would stay for dinner.

But usually Lane dined alone, to conserve her breath. Lane's live-in, John, served dinner on a TV tray beside her bed. She sat on the edge of the bed and leaned against a triangular pillow, where a heating pad brought relief to her painful back. On these evenings, she often complained. John, who would have just come home from work, hated to be criticized.

"You didn't close the refrigerator door this morning," Lane accused, as John brought in her dinner. "Yes I did," John replied, slamming down the tray. He wanted to take care of Lane, but he also wanted to be right.

The next day in my office, John said, "Lane and I live in the same house, but we can't seem to connect. She's always criticizing me." "Why don't you take the blame?" I suggested. "But I didn't do it," he answered. "That doesn't matter. Someone has to take the blame," I told him.

When John came home the next day, Lane said, "John, you forgot to fill the hummingbird feeder." He started to defend himself but then remembered my suggestion. With great reluctance, he said, "I'm sorry about that." For a moment he felt resentment fill his body like hot, black tar. Then he felt a sense of friendliness toward Lane. The exchange was like air going out of a balloon. "What did you do?" he heard himself ask Lane. "Susan filled it when she came at ten," she answered.

Suddenly John saw a frail little person waiting for him to get home, worried that he wouldn't come. What was he trying to defend? Lane's complaint of "If someone forgot to fill the feeder, would the birds go hungry?" might have masked a deeper concern: "What if someone forgot to change the oxygen?"

"How about a scotch and soda?" John asked Lane. "I thought you would never ask. My tongue is hanging out," she answered. John suggested she come out to the kitchen while he made the drink. Huffing and puffing, Lane walked to the kitchen and sat down at the table. "When you make a scotch and soda, fill the glass with ice cubes first, or you'll bruise the scotch," she ordered.

John felt a little flash of irritation. Then his resentment melted into humor. Bruise the scotch? He smiled and patted Lane on her shoulder as he put her drink down. Old people see our sorest, softest spots—the places where we get angry and impatient.

An elder is like your trainer, teaching you the lessons that you never learned from your mother. Or maybe it *is* your mother, trying one more time. She teaches you to go beyond the edge of who you think you are, what you thought you could do. With discipline you transform those narrow states of mind—the mind that criticizes, blames, and defends—into a light and spacious way of being, for yourself and for the elder in your care.

Late one afternoon my beeper went off as I drove home from work. John was going to be delayed at work, so I needed to stay with Lane for a while. When I arrived, Lane said she needed help walking to the bathroom. She stood up and struggled with her big metal walker. She'd take a step forward, stop, pant, rest, then pick up her walker again. It took Lane fifteen minutes to walk a hall I could have done in five seconds. I wanted her to hurry up. My body was with Lane, but my mind had long since reached the bathroom. My shoulders hunched over with impatience. Could my strong will force her forward faster?

Then in the midst of my distress, a ray of light flashed on the handle of the metal walker. Suddenly my mind and body came together. My mind slowed down to match the speed of a little body slowly walking down a long hall. I noticed a patch of peeling paint on the wall, heard the clatter of the walker tapping on the wood floor. "Wake up," I thought. "This vividness is enough."

CARE STUDY

Conflict and Well-Being

———◄o►———

Elizabeth lived alone in a little stone house with hardwood floors and scatter rugs. One night she tripped on a rug and broke her hip. Using her cane, Elizabeth pulled herself to the telephone. Help came, broke down the door, and took her to the hospital. After the break had mended, Elizabeth wanted her daughter to take care of her when she was released from the hospital, just as she had cared for her own mother.

"I can't take care of Mom," Bette told me as she paced back and forth in the hospital lobby. "Just because she took care of her mother for six years doesn't mean that I can care for her. My own kids need me now." That was the crux of the struggles that played themselves out over the next few years.

When Elizabeth found out that rather than going home with her daughter, she was going to have home care, she began raving. She complained about holes in the side of her house and how the hospital processed feces, then used conveyor belts to bring them down for dinner. "I'm a double person," she would yell, "a double-trouble person. Owwwww!" When a food technician at the hospital rolled a big metal cart into her room, Elizabeth screamed, "Get this metal out of my mouth."

Elizabeth still couldn't walk when she was released from the hospital. I was there with Bette when the ambulance attendants brought her into her house on a stretcher and transferred her to a rented hospital bed. Elizabeth was so distressed at the transition back home that she wet the bed.

Bette and I looked at each other. The trained helper would not arrive for two hours. Could we let Elizabeth lie there wet? Bette ran a hand through her short-cropped hair and pulled her ear. I looked down to see a piece of ice from my snow boot melting into the hardwood floor. Both of us probably thought of places we'd rather be. Then we started working together, figuring out how to change the bed with Elizabeth still in it.

As we worked, Elizabeth shouted, "You're killing me! Owwww! Mother, Mother!" In her confusion, she thought Bette was her mother. I thought of how, when I am sick, I, too, long for my mother. "Where are you when

I need you?" I think to myself. The longing to be someone's child does not die easily.

With all that chaos, what vivid recollections I still have: the sounds, the white sheets, the pink nightgown, the pot of brown-edged tulips we had brought home from the hospital. Finally, we tucked in the corners of the sheets and plumped up the pillow under Elizabeth's wiry little head, with its tufts of gray hair standing straight up. Bette finished buttoning up the top of her mother's flannel nightie. I brewed tea. Before long we sat sipping in satisfied silence. "What a fascinating world we've entered together," I thought.

That feeling of satisfaction didn't last long. The next day Elizabeth sat in her wheelchair and raved about evil people who came down the chimney to attack her in the night. She refused to let the couple who lived with her open the curtains in her hot, dark house. Her environment had become a mirror reflection of her bottomless depression.

"What kind of person was your mother before this accident happened?" I asked Bette. "She was a rugged pioneer type with an iron backbone," she told me. "She wouldn't talk about people or relationships. Mother shoveled coal. She knew the names of birds and flowers." Elizabeth had kept her yard, cleaned her house, and cared for her daughter.

Old now, with poor eyes and a broken hip, Elizabeth could no longer garden or clean, but she tried to cling to her identity as a mother. She wanted to be a mother and to be mothered. When Bette refused to take her in, Elizabeth felt so rejected, she broke down. Both her ability to do and her ability to be, in the only ways she had ever known, were gone. She had lost her ground. It was too much and too quick. She filled the emptiness with depression and hallucinated little children who thronged the house during the day and wailed in the night.

Elizabeth did not realize how times have changed and how changes in the economy have forced daughters as well as sons to go off to work. Bette was caught in a web of demands that left her scattered. Though Bette and Elizabeth were locked in struggle, we caregivers could not enter it. We might think that both women needed to expand their perspective, but we wouldn't say it out loud. Elizabeth's world was all we had to work with. We couldn't fight her false hopes; we only could trust that as her environment strengthened, she would give up her unrealistic views. Care proceeds not by resolving old conflicts but by creating an environment that expands the elder's world and promotes well-being.

Elizabeth had always been a fastidious person. Her closet was full of lovely clothes. But day after day, she sat around in her nightgown, depressed and growing smelly, refusing to take a bath. She reminded me of another old woman named Sharon.

One day Sharon's helper couldn't make it to work, so I went in her place. When I knocked on Sharon's door, she opened it a few inches and shouted, "Go away." Putting my foot in the door, I said to Sharon, "It's Ann. I've come to take care of you today." "I don't need help. Go away," she said. With my foot still in the door, I asked, "Excuse me, is that a Brooklyn accent?" When someone is cranky, you have to change the subject. That isn't always easy in such narrow circumstances, but it worked.

Sharon opened the door a few inches more and asked, "How did you know that?" "It was just a lucky guess," I replied. She looked me over and invited me in. "Do you want some tea?" she asked. After the tea I spoke to her directly: "I've come to give you a bath." "I don't want a bath," she answered, "and I'm not going to take one."

For a moment my hackles rose, and I became anxious that I might fail in my mission. Then I breathed in the conflict through the pores of my body until I quivered. I breathed out peace and clean smells and accomplishment. In and out I breathed, until we both relaxed.

"I'll draw the bathwater," I said. "Do you want some of that bubble bath your daughter sent you?" "No, bubbles make me sneeze," she responded. I waited, thinking she had forgotten why I had come, until she finally said, "It's good to be clean." I hurried into the bathroom and started the water running. Then, before she could withdraw her consent, I lowered Sharon gently into the warm water.

After washing her back and letting her relax in the water awhile, I wrapped Sharon in a warm towel, dried her off, and helped her dress. As I opened the curtains to let in the late morning light, Sharon rolled her eyes to heaven. With me right there in the room, she began to pray: "Dear Lord in heaven, please protect me from this woman. Only you know how her mind works. Amen."

I breathed in the insult. Had I exerted too much power over this fragile woman? I wondered. Why didn't she appreciate my attempts to help? Why do I always want to feel appreciated? Then I switched and breathed out practicality. Did it matter if I was too powerful or underappreciated? I breathed out trust in myself while I brushed Sharon's hair.

Now Elizabeth, too, was remembering that she valued cleanliness. "It's not good to be dirty," she said. Taking this as consent, her helper and I bathed Elizabeth, dressed her, opened the curtains, and watched her preen in front of the mirror.

One day Elizabeth found an old diary. She could not believe that she was the person who had written it. As she woke up to what she had become, she got enraged, and her rage pushed her helpers to go further. We had to ask ourselves, "Who is this person? What has she been in life?" We remembered that Elizabeth's strength had been her independence. Perhaps we could support that independence. Elizabeth had grown stronger, but she had become too dependent on her helpers. "Don't leave me alone," she would yell if the helper went into the kitchen to prepare a meal. We decided to cut back her level of care so she would have afternoons alone.

We started out slowly, with Elizabeth having thirty minutes by herself. She complained, but we left her sitting at her dining room table with a cup of tea. Inches away was the telephone, and right beside it, written large, were the phone numbers of three people who could be called in the event of an emergency. Elizabeth was so proud of herself for having half an hour alone that we extended the time to one hour, then two hours, and finally four. She learned to cherish her independence, and for two years she kept to that schedule.

As Elizabeth became frailer with age, she again got stuck in the idea that her daughter should be the one to take care of her. Finally, money became the decisive factor in this mother-daughter struggle. Elizabeth was eighty-eight, her money was dipping lower, and Bette was tired of running back and forth from her town to her mother's. She decided to put Elizabeth into a nursing home close to her house.

I drove over to tell Elizabeth good-bye. She lay on her bed wailing and raving. "Bette is coming to take you to the nursing home," I told her. "She wants you to be close to her." "That's what I want," said Elizabeth, suddenly rational. Then she went back to wailing. Soon after Elizabeth went to the nursing home, she died, happily, with her daughter at her side.

*

There are conflicts in our lives for which there are no solutions: differences in temperament, needs, timing, rhythm, and pace. But a circle of care goes forward anyway, stoking the fires, providing nourishment and friendship, and helping everyone do what has to be done.

CARE STUDY

Delusions and Relaxation

————◄o►————

Dick was a large man, with a high forehead and a long Roman nose, an oil man who had traveled the world building business empires and watching them crumble. He had known love, but at ninety-two he looked back on his marriages as "mistake number one and mistake number two." His second marriage had ended when he was eighty-five.

His second wife, younger and trying her best to control Dick's physical and mental health, had put him on a strict diet and a tight budget. But Dick could not give up his wild, entrepreneurial ways. His expansive self-image had been unable to endure the limitations of old age. In his loneliness he visualized himself as an entrepreneur roaming the world, building one success after another. His love of gambling led him to fall prey to swindlers who sent him offers in the mail. "Congratulations, you've won a new car," one letter said. "All you have to do is send fifty dollars." Before long Dick was spending several hundred dollars a month trying to win prizes. He pictured himself driving up to an oil rig in a new car that he had just won, with a million dollars in the bank and a pretty girl at his side.

One day a crook called him at home and talked him into giving out his bank account number. The thief made off with several thousand dollars. Dick's wife, in frustration, took away his checkbook. He thus lost both his dignity and his source of entertainment. Before long he began to hallucinate happier days in the oil fields, and his wife left him. Barely able to see, Dick ended up alone in a hotel. He offered big tips to those who attended to his needs. It was the only way he knew to make himself feel important.

His grandchildren, remembering him as a knight in shining armor, rented him an apartment in the city where they lived, so they could care for him. I was there with the grandchildren when Dick was brought to his new apartment. As we plumped up the pillows under his head, Dick looked up at me and said, "Thank you, Bob. Now let's take down that rig."

Dick dwelled in the realm of his mind. He lived in his dreams and ignored the rest. Dick had only connected to the successes in his life, never to the times in between. His image of himself as an oil man was of someone who was above the ordinary concerns of domestic life or relationships. He didn't seem to remember the times when what he'd built had crumbled. The doctor called him senile; he sometimes responded to voices that only he could hear. He didn't relate to his caregivers as individuals; he called everyone Bob.

If he got the slightest glimmer that someone didn't go along with his way of thinking, Dick became angry. He seemed to put out invisible feelers to check for responses. He knew he wasn't in an oil field, but he ignored that. He used anger as a way to keep helpers from challenging him. Once he said, "I'm going to sit here and shout until you give me what I want."

Dick was severely stooped, he could barely walk, and he often lost his balance. He refused to do any exercise. He spent his days watching television and dreaming of going back to work. Sometimes we wanted to shout at him, "Dick, you're ninety-two, and you're not ever going back to work. Do your exercises. Get used to being old." But we didn't.

Too often, when we see elements of denial in old people, we want to cut through by shouting or otherwise "setting them straight." We want to lecture them on self-improvement and psychological health. These methods, which we've all used at one time or another, only alienate people.

Dick suffered from an affliction that besets many of us in this culture, albeit in a milder form. We are so attached to the doing of our lives that we forget to simply be. As a society, we're always "pumping it up." We dwell on beginnings and try to forget endings. We display our happiness and try to cover up our sadness. We encounter a stoplight but continue jogging in place, desperately trying to keep our heart rate up.

But we can't always be up. What about the times when we feel no inspiration, no energy? We can learn to appreciate ourselves during low times as well as high times. We can walk a middle road, where our self-image is synchronized with the reality of the present moment. It is a big task, but it will help us overcome denial in old age.

When a person at the end of a relationship, a job, or a life pretends that nothing has ended, that nothing has been lost, he is living in the fog of denial. Denial begins when someone disowns present-day reality and lives in the memory of what he did many years ago. Anything that interferes with this imagined life is shut out, maybe by drinking excessively or by staying alone with the curtains closed or by surrounding himself with admirers.

Sometimes caregivers or family members feed the elder's denial; they may want to support the elder's delusions because they're afraid she'll feel sad or hopeless or that she'll die and leave them. If a person's denial is supported by family and friends, a caregiver must paddle skillfully through those muddy waters. If the caregiver supports the denial, the care won't be healing. If she tries to confront the denial head-on, she'll run into opposition. If a husband insists that his aged wife wear high-heeled shoes to support his fantasy of still being young and the wife obliges, you might judge her for giving in to her husband's fantasy. But never make the mistake of taking sides in such a conflict. Instead, expand your own view. Look at the fifty-year marriage between this man and woman, appreciate their endurance, and inquire how their relationship works. The bonds between child and parent, between husband and wife, even between giver and receiver of care are deeper than our surface judgments can fathom. If you look at these bonds with an unbiased mind, you will see an opening where denial can begin to be nudged a little toward acknowledgment.

Instead of focusing on the denial, work more on introducing connecting activities that expand the world surrounding the old person. Brighten the space around the ignoring, so that the present environment becomes more attractive. Dick visualized old times because he could see no happiness in his present circumstances. Nights were hell for him and his helpers. As soon as daylight faded, he became forgetful. He itched all over. He'd call out, "Bob, Bob, put some lotion on my skin. Bring me a drink. Bring me toilet paper. I need a woman." Sometimes he dreamed he was on a hot-air balloon and running out of steam. Sometimes he was about to fall from an oil rig, or he was running from a gush of hot oil through an underground pipe.

The fading of day and the blackness of night reminded him of death and failure. One evening I went to see him. "I'm a zero. I'm a zero. I'm a zero," he said to me. "You mean you're back to square one?" I asked. "No," he said, "I missed my goal, and I'm nowhere." We listened with empathy to Dick's misery over his unfulfilled longings.

For an old person, how the evening goes is the biggest factor in whether the night will be restful or hellish. So Dick's helpers and his grandchildren worked together to cheer up his evenings. On a typical evening, his helper Phil cooked a meal in the kitchen while Dick sat in his chair in the living room. Phil put on some music, set the table with colorful place mats and dishes, and put a bowl of yellow flowers in the center. One of the grandchildren arrived, and he and Dick drank apple juice while dinner cooked.

After supper the grandson helped Phil put Dick to bed. "I don't want to go to bed," Dick protested. "Yeah, we know," the two men said as they slipped off his clothes. They rubbed lotion on his skin, buttoned up his pajamas, and walked him to his chair. The grandson left, and Dick and Phil watched a program on television. Then Phil helped Dick to bed and played his guitar for a few minutes as Dick drifted into sleep.

Usually Dick would wake before morning. "Bob, Bob," he'd cry out, "I'm itching all over. Get me some lotion. Get me down from this rig." But over time he relaxed more, stayed asleep longer, and was able to recount his dreams. Once he dreamed he was at his high school prom and had lost his clothes. He woke up shaking the bars of his bed. Another night he dreamed that as he was returning from work, his car fell out from under him.

The circle of care stayed steady through Dick's ups and downs. The members of the team focused on making the environment cheerful and dependable. They kept their attention focused on the practical details of care. In this way they helped Dick to return home from the oil fields at last and get ready to die.

Desires, Demands, and Boundaries

One day I was sitting in my office when the phone rang. "I need a drink," a gruff voice told me over the phone. It was Harriet, a seventy-five-year-old woman of beauty, wealth, and talent. When Harriet was eighteen, her parents, unable to handle their creative and outrageous child, had put her in a straitjacket and sent her off to an insane asylum.

For more than fifty years, Harriet had spent several months each year drinking and getting increasingly disruptive and violent, followed by several months drying out in the hospital. She had lived her life, which included a short marriage and the death of her son, shuttling between her luxurious high-rise apartment and a mental institution. Harriet had never realized her talents or helped others. She trusted no one, least of all herself.

On some days, Harriet ran around her apartment throwing out all the food, smoking several cigarettes at once, and attacking anyone in sight. On other days, she could barely be aroused from deep sleep, too depressed even to smoke.

It was Bill Brauer, the director of our agency, who came up with a creative plan for Harriet's care. He told me that when people have strong desires, you can use them as a tool to help them. He went to see Harriet and worked out her plan of care. They agreed that she could have two drinks per day, under the following conditions: she had to have the drinks at five o'clock; she had to be sitting in the living room; she had to eat at least three canapés with the drinks; and she had to eat a regular dinner later. Harriet wanted to drink, so she agreed to these conditions.

You might question a care plan that includes serving drinks to an alcoholic. But instead of judging the woman's desire, the strategy was to appreciate it and bring to it a sense of boundary. The plan uplifted the space around the desire.

This kind of plan only works when there is twenty-four-hour care. The helpers watched the time, so that Harriet would not forget when five o'clock came. The hors d'oeuvres were specially prepared with her favorite delicacies. Harriet did not want a big bottle of vodka in the house, so each day her helper brought a tiny bottle. While Harriet drank, dinner was prepared. The aroma of good cooking filled the apartment. "Do you think there is still hope for me?" Harriet asked, as she sat down to her meal. The caregivers were becoming her allies rather than her watchdogs.

But as the friendships strengthened, Harriet began to show her fear of the intimacy. Underlying her desire to drink was a desire, based on fear, to avoid becoming too intimate with others. The more Harriet's health improved, the more she began to act up. Some days Harriet would call the office and complain to Bill Brauer. "I don't know why I can't get a decent meal in this house," she raged. She was not eating anything. She would throw the food on the floor or at the helpers. The care plan didn't seem to be working anymore.

Bill decided to invite Harriet to come to the office for a meeting of the care team so she could air her complaints. As soon as Harriet arrived, Bill said, "Now, Harriet, home care is different from hospital care. It's your house, not an institution. We want to make sure that we're doing things the way you like them done. How is it going?" "Oh, just fine," Harriet replied.

"How about the food, Harriet? Do you like the food?" Bill asked. "Yes, that's the best thing. Every day the girls make me a gourmet dinner." Everyone on the team was startled to see that Harriet dropped her anger as soon as she was included as a member of the team. Her new plan of care encouraged interaction with the world beyond her apartment.

Soon Harriet got cancer. She had to go to the hospital each day for treatments. It was decided that she should not be taken in an ambulance; instead, she would get dressed and go in a taxi, as a means of increasing her opportunity for interaction.

So every day Harriet went to the hospital and sat in the waiting room. Noticing children with cancer waiting their turn broadened Harriet's mind beyond her own troubles. "I want to buy toys for them," she said. She never did—but just the intention was enough to induce a more peaceful state of mind.

*

The most important aspect of the caregiving team is having the flexibility to embrace changing circumstances. Then desires and demands become gateways. An old habit can propel both elder and caregivers into a more cheerful manner of being. In this way, the helped becomes the helper, the helper the helped, and the boundaries between them fall away.

CHAPTER 9

————◄o►————

Respite Care and the Nursing Home

M ANY ELDERS, SOONER OR LATER, will require more care than their families can provide in the home setting and will need some form of assisted living or nursing home. Sometimes the move away will be temporary, to allow the elder to recover from an illness or to allow the caregivers to rest. Other times it will be permanent. When a loved one must have twenty-four-hour care for whatever reason, and there is not enough money to provide that care in the home, then a nursing home is the solution. This chapter discusses the important steps in making that transition.

REALIZING WHEN YOU NEED HELP

An important part of effective, loving caregiving is realizing when you need a break or more long-term help. The strain and hard work of caring for an elderly person can cause caregivers to burn out. I don't mean merely short-term fatigue. If you're simply tired or emotionally drained, you can recover by resting. The burnout I'm referring to is more serious; it comes from living with unrelieved stress. You feel a little sick, but you don't go to the doctor. You feel a little pain, but you ignore it. You just keep going, not sleeping enough and not eating well. You have put the details of your own life on hold indefinitely to spend all your energy tending to the needs of others. A kind of depression develops, and you lose your joy in living.

Often the first step in helping a loved one make the transition to a nursing home environment is to acknowledge your own attitudes so you can quit fighting yourself. Do you doubt whether using a nursing home is the right approach? Then the elder, too, will be full of doubt. Clarity is the antidote for doubt, so try and get matters clear in your own mind. Confidence comes when you can accept what is, not with regret but with calm, as a challenge to go forward. Sometimes you have to say, "Putting mother in a home is the worst thing I ever had to do." Sometimes you listen to the elder say, "This is the worst thing that ever happened to me." Then you can cheer up and be with the circumstances of your life without phony optimism.

My father spent a little over a year in a nursing home. After a year of living with my sister and five months in the hospital, he had gone back to live with his wife, Eleanor. He had a caregiver with him during the day while she was at work, but after a while it became clear that he needed more care than we could provide at home. He moved into the nursing home that was right next door to their apartment. On my visits to California, I had often walked past this building of pink adobe surrounded by grass and trees. I had always been attracted to its appearance, but I had never gone in.

As soon as my father moved to the nursing home, I went to California to spend two weeks with him. Before I could be of help to him, I had to face my own sense of failure and guilt that my father had to live in a nursing home. As I sat beside his bed, I felt completely bankrupt. I wanted to lie down and weep.

Then I thought about a friend of mine, who had been able to keep her mother at home with twenty-four-hour care. The care was working beautifully, but my friend confided to me that she felt so guilty that she wasn't personally taking care of her mother. She cried buckets of tears that she could not hold her mother as she had been held as a baby. My friend and I both suffered from a belief that a family is a closed unit.

As I thought of my father and my friend, gradually my sense of balance was restored. "Let's walk," my father said. He used his walker, and we strolled out into the hall and around the home. While I followed my father's schedule of walking and resting, walking and resting, I let myself absorb the atmosphere in the home. I began to see the threads of connection in the midst of the confusion. I saw that my determined father was happy, because he had a goal of trying to get well and he saw Eleanor every day.

As I began to make friends with some of the other residents and staff, I got a sense of the rhythm of life that was going on around my father. After a time my perspective changed. I could begin to explore the possibilities within the immediate environment of the nursing home.

A nursing home can be the heartbreak hotel at the end of a lonely street, or it can be a nourishing source of community for a frail elder. Group living can be good for some people. The stereotype of old people sitting around under bright lights, on linoleum floors, in their wheelchairs is no longer true of most nursing homes. As with home caregiving, those who love the elder can do much to ensure the success of this new way of living.

CHOOSING A NURSING HOME

Before you begin exploring nursing homes, I would suggest that you read an excellent book on the subject: *Old Friends*, by Tracy Kidder. It gives you a complete look at nursing home life from the inside out. It shows that the dignity of life, what is essential in an ordinary way, can be continued and even learned within the nursing-home environment.

In general, around the country, there are four levels of care offered for older people. A nursing home may combine several levels of care. Level one, the skilled nursing home, offers a complete range of skilled nursing and other rehabilitative services as well as recreational activities. There is usually a limit on the amount of time that insurance will pay for skilled care. For instance, after surgery or a broken hip, insurance may pay for a given number of days in a skilled nursing home for further recovery and rehabilitative services, such as physical therapy or occupational therapy. When the person has recovered as much as he can, he may go back home or into the longer-term care of level two. Level two also provides nursing care, but the expectation is that the person will take a long time to recover or will not be able to recover. He will perhaps need care for the rest of his life. Insurance does not usually cover level two care unless your parent has long-term care insurance. Then there is the third level: assisted living or board-and-care homes, which are also called group homes, sheltered housing, residential care homes, and adult congregate living homes. Assisted living provides meals, some help with personal care and housekeeping, and may or may not include activities. Level three offers nursing supervision or overview but not direct nursing. In level four, meals are offered but no nursing supervision.

More and more skilled nursing homes that offer twenty-four-hour skilled nursing and other rehabilitative services are becoming temporary dwellings, providing people who have received intensive treatment in a hospital with a place in which to receive further treatment before returning home. Levels two and three both may offer temporary stays for older people as well, so the family can have respite for a few days, weeks, or even months.

When choosing a nursing home or other respite-care home, consider what your particular need is. If your mother has had surgery, she may need skilled nursing for a while to recover. Perhaps your father is taking a course of treatment such as chemotherapy and needs a protected environment close to the hospital where the treatment is being given. Does your mother need intensive rehabilitation following a broken hip? Does your family need a summer off from taking care of your father so you can focus more on your teenage child? Do you want to bring your mother to live near you? Or does your mother want to stay within her own community but can't afford the cost of the twenty-four-hour care that she needs to stay in her own home? Does your parent suffer from dementia and need more skilled intervention than you feel you can provide? Once you have defined your own need, it will help you narrow down your search and enable you to assess the nursing home or assisted-living dwelling with far greater clarity.

In your local bookstore or on the Internet, you can find many books that provide extensive checklists of things to look for in a nursing home or an assisted-living dwelling. But finding a place you're comfortable with goes beyond lists of questions to ask. The intangibles—the attitude and atmosphere of the home—are of equal or greater importance. They can also be the most difficult to grasp. When you first consider a nursing home, you are on the outside looking in. What you have to do as best you can is get a feel for what it is like from the inside looking out. This may take a while.

Regard the nursing home or assisted-living situation as a way to extend and enrich the elder's world. And look for a place where the family and the professionals can work together in the same way that you would do in the home-care setting.

Location, as with real estate, is key. If possible, try to find a nursing home close to a family member. One reason nursing-home care worked for my father is that his wife visited him every day. His nursing home was about three hundred yards from the front door of his apartment, one block from his church, a block from his little neighborhood shopping center. And it was only about six blocks from where Eleanor worked. It was in a neighborhood in which he had lived for twenty years. Although he had become disconnected from many aspects of his life and from his image of himself, he was able to reconnect through relationships with many new people who extended his feeling of community and connection.

People often ask, "Should I leave my parents in their old neighborhood, or should I bring them into mine?" There is no set answer to that question, but whichever neighborhood you choose, there has to be a connective link—a spouse, son, daughter, grandchild, or care coordinator who helps the elder reestablish his or her life and reconnect to what has been disconnected. If a very old person moves into a new neighborhood, it will take effort to connect to a new life.

Settling In

A move into a group living situation generally creates a big break in a person's life journey. The move, in itself difficult, may bring a feeling of disconnection from an environment that had been a source of strength for many years. Usually some trauma has necessitated the move. Exhaustion and fear on the part of the elder and the family are likely at this time. The elder has probably lost the identity of mother, father, businessperson, or teacher. Now it's time for this person to find out who he or she is apart from the roles once played in life. When life's work ceases, can old people just be? Can we help them find simple being?

It is easy for a person to lose his sense of ground when he moves into a new home. The task for the family is to help the elder find his sense of place within the new environment. Most nursing homes are sensitive to the difficulty of moving in. A social worker or an activity director may assist with orientation. Sometimes there is a resident committee that helps newcomers get established. A family member can help to ease the way, or the family can hire a caregiver for a day or two to go through the new routines of daily living with the elder. He has to become familiar with his new room, where his possessions are kept, the meal service, and how to get around to find the various activities. He will be making new relationships with other residents and staff, and it takes time for people to trust one another.

Visit the nursing home at different times of day—during activities and at mealtimes. Sit in the dining room, the lobby, and the elder's room. Help the elder walk up and down the halls. Don't judge; just observe. You're learning how the home works in order to bring more clarity into your own mind.

Good physical support will help to relax the mind. The first task is to pay attention to the room. Everyone's room should hold some favorite and familiar items. Some old people have forgotten their preferences or how to express them, so other people may have to uncover them. My father had yellow pads and pencils on his table so he could get up early and write, and he had a little boom box and tapes so he could listen to music. He also had a few framed family photos. The main thing is to work with the available space to make it attractive, functional, and nourishing.

Bring in favorite colors. Make sure the chair fits the space and is comfortable. Make sure the bedspread is attractive and the fabric is pleasant to the touch. The paintings on the wall should be ones that have meaning for the elder. Something from home is nice, if it harmonizes with the room. In a small space, every object will be significant. Keep the room simple and to the elder's liking.

Hair care is another important issue. Women especially want a becoming and easy style as well as a mirror in which to see themselves. Find out whether the nursing assistant will fix the elder's hair for her or whether there is a hairdresser who comes to the home. If she can still go out to the hairdresser, who will take her? There was a barber in my father's nursing home, but Eleanor took my father out to his favorite barber to have his hair cut. Make sure the elder's clothes are attractive and fit well, just as you would at home.

In every way you can, make the environment pleasing to the sight, the touch, and the taste, and let it resonate to the beat of life. Make the room and the person stand out like shining stars.

Find out about activities in the home. Can the elder take part? Maybe you can help out in some way. Most nursing homes really need and value volunteer help, and residents gain status when their spouses or children are around. Volunteer to lead a session on current events, with the person you care for at your side; explain interesting news items, and ask easy questions. Volunteer to serve refreshments at a group discussion. Participate in exercises in the morning, call a game of bingo, or volunteer to lead a group sing-along or a ladies' tea followed by nail polishing.

Let yourself go slowly. It takes a while to connect to the good times in a nursing home. Participate in the games, go on the walks, help with the trips to the park. Attend the concerts. Sit in the lobby and look at people in wheelchairs talking to family or one another. Notice the sun as it shines through imperfectly washed windows. Even if the atmosphere is claustrophobic, stay awhile. If you don't run away, you will find your heart opening to the real life around you.

Supporting a Person in a Nursing Home

For the nursing-home experience to be a good one, the family has to work hand in hand with the staff in the same way they would with home care. Don't take the attitude that you are abandoning a loved one to a nursing home; see it instead as opening up the family unit. All of us, young or old, need to feel that we are connected, that we care and share responsibility for one another.

The family can help lift the spirits of the elder by supporting and encouraging friendships with other residents. My father made good friends while he was in the nursing home, both with some of the professional staff and with two other residents. The family promoted these friendships by taking one of the friends with my father when he walked down to the corner to have a Coke every evening and by inviting the friends to watch videos with my father. The family paid special attention to the friends when they came for concerts and church services.

It is a challenge for many families to receive help from others. Opening up the family unit may bring to light unresolved conflicts that are painful to look at. Many family members stay away from the nursing home because visits bring up emotional pain. Seeing a loved one in a nursing home may evoke broken dreams of what the family could have been, before it was scattered to the winds. It may help to attend a support group or an educational group for families, which many good nursing homes offer.

The problems that come up in nursing homes often involve communication difficulties. If residents, staff, and families don't communicate well with one another, misunderstandings proliferate. This happens easily in a nursing home, where so many people with so many needs coexist in such a small space. Many families are afraid that if they express their concerns to the management, there will be reprisals against the elder.

It helps to learn the lines of communication within the home. Are there regular conferences between the professional staff and the family? To whom do you talk if you have concerns about personal care, medications, or food? If you express concerns to an aide, will he communicate them to the nurse, social worker, or activity director?

If the elder is driving the nursing-home personnel crazy hunting for her underwear every morning, remember that very few staff members are likely to be stealing it, no matter what the elder may say. Find out why the elder is running out of clean underwear. Maybe she needs more sets to last from one laundering to the next. Or maybe the laundry system is poorly organized. What can be done?

Although my father was in a good nursing home, some typical difficulties came up during the course of his care. For instance, he had a poor relationship with a man who worked the evening shift, a nurse with an authoritarian style. My father couldn't stand to have anyone tell him what to do. When the nurse did so, my father told everyone that the nurse had tripped him and made him fall. We couldn't disregard what my father was saying, and he did have a bruise, but it seemed unlikely that the nurse had tripped him. Eleanor set up a meeting with my father and the nurse, and an understanding was established. My father stopped accusing the nurse, and their relationship improved. The important point is to keep an open mind and to nurture relationships by communicating directly.

Another way to uplift spirits is to take the elder for an outing. Sometimes a family is afraid to take an elder out for fear that he won't want to return. That wasn't true with my father, who always wanted to go back. He just needed to feel part of the larger community. Home visits, visiting family, and taking a drive out of town are all good ways to cheer someone up. Eleanor took my father to a mall every Saturday so he could walk around and have lunch at a restaurant.

If the elder is too frail to go out, the celebrations can be brought to the nursing home. Look especially for opportunities to bring young children for a visit. Has a grandson done a drawing that he's proud of? Save it to show grandmother. Does a granddaughter have her Halloween costume or birthday party dress all picked out? Bring the youngster over in the afternoon to show the elder. There's nothing like a child to bring the breath of life into a nursing home. The elder and everyone else on the floor will appreciate it.

But you don't have to do much of anything to uplift the spirits of the elder. Just relax and be with what is happening. Get a Coke; hear the sizzle as you pour it over ice. As you listen to an old song coming from the room next door, relax and feel the words and music. Open your eyes and look around. Your spirits will lift and spread.

CHAPTER 10

———◄○►———

The Generosity of the Dying

I SPOKE WITH MY FATHER on the phone the day before he died. It was his eightieth birthday, and he and Eleanor were at my sister's house. My other sister was there, too, so it was a family celebration. My father had a bad cold and wasn't feeling well, but I had no idea that he was close to death.

As I started to say good-bye, I suddenly told him that I loved him and that I would soon be in California to spend time with him. There was a long silence. Then he answered, "Your book, when are you going to get your book finished?" I said that I was working away on it, but it was taking longer than I thought. "It always does," he said, as he hung up the phone.

When my sister called me the next morning to tell me that he had died, my mind couldn't quite grasp it. Even though my father had been an invalid for a long time, a part of me believed his own notion that he was invincible.

When I reflected back on that last conversation with my father, I thought of his silence when I had told him I would see him in the summer. Did he know, with the prescience of the dying, that we would not see each other again? I wondered if we had left any unfinished business. At first I regretted that his last words to me were about my work, but then I realized that that was his generosity.

The face of love my father always presented to me was one of practicality. His father had given him a family coat of arms that proclaimed, "Aspire, persevere, and indulge not." My father's vision had led him toward expansion of his ideas and his business, sometimes unrealistically, but always with a good heart. Even though my aspirations have taken me down different paths from his, the coat of arms hangs on my wall, along with pictures of other teachers who have taught me to wear family heritage as a badge of honor.

In my work with people who are dying, I try to help families receive the many faces of love that their loved one reveals: passionate love, parental love, brotherly love, practical love, expansive love, overprotective love. Sometimes the love connection is explosive, bursting out like fireworks with anger and wounds to the heart. Receiving the generosity of the dying person entails looking and listening and trusting the different faces of love.

Use all of your senses, feelings, and intuition to look below the surface, accepting that sometimes love shows itself in odd and hidden ways. Get in touch with your tenderness and let it shine out. Then the dignity of the elder's life will become a guide for everyone.

SIGNPOSTS OF DYING

Physical signs of dying are the easiest ones to see. The person's arms and legs may become cool to the touch, and the back may become darker in color. He or she may become incontinent of urine and feces. Oral secretions may become more profuse and collect in the back of the throat, as the result of the inability to cough up or swallow the saliva that is normally produced. Eyesight may fade as well as hearing.

You might notice that the elder has less interest in what is going on in the immediate environment. Sometimes he begins to give away his possessions. An old woman with a runny nose may not relate to the box of tissues at her side, right where it has always been; she will wait passively until someone wipes her nose. The elder's interest in family and caregivers may also diminish: a son who comes to visit his mother may ask how she's feeling and she doesn't answer.

The body may seem to be a burden, with the elder able to walk only a few steps before getting tired. Sometimes she will gradually spend more and more time sleeping during the day, and it may become increasingly difficult to wake her up. You may notice a change in the breathing pattern during sleep. There may be very short periods of no breathing. This is called apnea and is the result of decreased circulation and buildup of body wastes. The desire and need for food and drink may diminish.

Many people who are dying become increasingly confused about time, place, and the identity of familiar people. Many have visions that others cannot see, sometimes of loved ones who have gone before. They may become restless, as a result of decreased circulation of oxygen to the brain.

Sometimes—oddly—there may be outer signs of inner agitation. The elder may sit quietly doing nothing, but his inner chaos may show in the external environment—the dog will yap, the fire alarm will go off accidentally. The environment crackles and pops, as old attachments snap. Sometimes the elder may be sitting quietly, but the helper experiences the agitation within herself.

Good days and bad days may alternate. Some days the elder may get up, look out the window, comment on the beautiful day, eat a good breakfast, and want to see a friend. The next day when he gets up, he might stare into space for two hours and then take a nap. Caregivers are never sure what to expect, which can throw them off balance.

An elder may show you in an oblique way that she is expecting death. One woman I know who is approaching the end of her life thinks that all the flowers in her living room are white tulips, even though they are roses and peonies. The family knows that white tulips are an image of death and renewal to their mother: she once planted white tulips when her infant son died.

Remember, life and death are mysterious. A person might die with no warning, with none of these signposts—and any of these signs might appear with the elder still years away from death.

Supporting the Dying Person

When a person is dying, the support needs to start on the physical level, to bring as much comfort as possible. If someone is dying at home, pay special attention to her preferred place to sit or lie down. Many people would rather lie on a sofa or in a reclining chair. You can rent a hospital bed and set it up in the living room. The important point is to allow the place to be chosen by the elder, if at all possible.

Ask the doctor whether the elder could have hospice care. Hospice is an organization that provides care for the dying by strengthening the supportive environment. When a physician refers a patient to hospice, he is saying that there is no cure for the patient's condition, that the dying person has six months or less to live. The goal for treatment then becomes what is called palliative care, which is bringing comfort to the dying person through symptom relief and pain control and working to create a caring environment that includes not only the needs of the dying person but those of the family as well.

The focus of the hospice and palliative care approach is to help the person live as fully as possible during whatever time remains. The care is provided by a team that includes a physician, nurses, the family, social workers, chaplains, bereavement counselors, and volunteers. Sometimes home health aides are provided. When the doctor makes a referral, hospice will do an assessment to determine the care needs of the elder as well as the needs of the family. They will familiarize the family or primary caregiver and the patient with the hospice philosophy and guidelines and help them to accept that the care has become palliative rather than curative.

One advantage to hospice care is that a hospice nurse is available for consultation twenty-four hours a day. The hospice nurse will also make periodic visits to help the primary caregiver with treatments, training, and administering medications. Hospice will provide visits from a social worker, a physical therapist, and a chaplain. A personal-care attendant will come from once to several times a week or even daily, according to the assessed need. A volunteer will be assigned to help in a neighborly way by running errands, making friendly visits, and perhaps doing some respite care so the primary caregiver can have a rest.

Medicare and Medicaid and most insurances will pay for hospice care. Medicare has a hospice benefit. However, if the family needs to hire a primary caregiver or extra care beyond what hospice provides, then that cost would not be covered by insurance. So when the assessment is performed, it is important to get clear about what costs will be involved.

Most hospice care is given within the home. Some hospitals also have special hospice units to attend to the medical aspects of a person's dying or to provide respite for family members who need relief. Sometimes people think that if they sign up for hospice, they cannot go to the hospital, but that is not the case. The hospice benefit allows days in the hospital for treatments and for respite for the family. And a person can revoke her hospice benefit at any time if she changes her mind and wants to try for a cure again.

In addition to physical support, it is helpful to look at the whole environment of care to see what is needed. Sometimes this means attending to the elder's partner or family as well as to the elder himself. I once consulted with the children of a very frail man who was being cared for by his second wife. The children were upset that his meals were inadequate and that occasionally the wife left home and didn't return for several days. They saw how grieved their father was at his wife's absence. Yet when caregivers were hired to take care of the father, the wife would come back and get rid of the helpers. This pattern repeated itself over and over. The family didn't know what to do to keep their father safe. Should they bring him home with them? Should they move him into a nursing home?

In a consultation with the husband and wife, she said, "I don't want to leave him alone, but I have to go back to my other house and check to see if it is all right. Someone might have broken in. Maybe my possessions have been stolen." What the wife was really saying was, "I'm afraid my husband is dying. I have to get away." She badly needed a helper.

Finally, the wife agreed to have personal care for her husband, even though she was there in the house. A care coordinator went frequently to the house and began to establish a relationship with the wife, using her husband's care as a means to communicate with her. After the relationship became established, the care coordinator was able to bring in a few more helpers—someone to clean the house, someone to take the wife shopping. Eventually, the coordinator took the wife to a caregiver support group, which provided transportation as well as help looking after her husband while she was gone. By caring for the primary caregiver, the caregiving team enabled the dying man to get what he needed.

COMMUNICATING WITH THE DYING PERSON

It is necessary to establish trust with someone who is dying. One element of trustworthiness is telling the truth. Dying people need to be told that they are dying, and they need a chance to process their feelings about it. Because of my work, the subject of death has always been familiar around my house. Maybe I overdid it with my son. When he was four, we visited a frail friend in a nursing home. As soon as we sat down with her, my son asked her politely, "When are you going to die?" My friend laughed and told him, "Not right now." Good communication about dying requires a little more sensitivity than just using the word.

When someone has a terminal illness, it is important to sit with her and acknowledge the impending death. Often a person who is dying will apologize for being in bed. "I don't know why I'm so tired!" she might say. The helper can gently tell her the truth: "I'm sorry you aren't feeling well. Maybe it's because of your lung cancer." One very frail old man, about to undergo brain surgery, kept looking at me in a meaningful way. I took his hand. "Are you worried that you won't live through this operation?" I asked. "I'm afraid I won't make it," he said. He gave me a searching look, and I confirmed that indeed he might not live through it. We were very close at that moment. We trusted each other, and because of that trust, we relaxed.

For so many in our society, the subject of death is delicate and brings up fear. If someone suffers from extreme confusion or fear, direct communication might be hard. You know that if you don't tell the truth, you will not have been helpful. But if you do tell the truth, you may have to deal with difficult repercussions. You may be able to sit down and say, "Mom, I'm afraid you're going to die soon," but you don't know whether she comprehends your words. If she is very fearful, she might react to your honesty with anger or with unusual behavior.

Lavina was a lovely lady who lived in a split-level house with champagne-colored carpets and modern art on the walls. She had a hopeless liver condition. Lavina's son asked me to be the one to tell his mother that she didn't have long to live. Lavina lay in her modern bedroom in the middle of a king-size bed. Her nervous fingers pulled the blanket up to her chin, rolled it down, pulled it up, and rolled it down again.

After we had talked for a while, I told Lavina that I had spoken to her doctor. She asked me what he had said. I told her that her liver was failing and that, much to my regret, she did not have many days left. "Bonnie dropped a jar of mustard on my new blue carpet," she responded. I told Lavina that I thought the caregiver had been nervous and moving too quickly. "I'm going to sue you," she said. I told Lavina that I was sorry her liver was failing and that I wanted to help her in any way that I could. "Well, get Bonnie out of here. She's a clumsy girl," she replied.

With that, Lavina got up from her bed, got in her car, and drove away. For three days, she ran around town shopping, playing bridge, and going to movies, until she could go no further. At that point, Bonnie and I took her to the doctor's office, and he put her in the hospital. Her son came from out of town. He told her, "Mother, I wish it weren't true, but you're going to die soon." "I'm ready," she said. "I've done all I can." That night she died peacefully.

Some people accept their dying as an ordinary event. When Cyrus was seventy, he met a spiritual teacher and moved to Boulder, Colorado, to study and practice meditation. He was alone in the world, without wife or children. As time passed, the Buddhist community became his family. Volunteers were coordinated to help him with shopping and housework. Members of the community gave him rides to events and frequently invited him to dinner. Cyrus rarely missed a community meeting or major practice session. While others sat on cushions on the floor, Cyrus sat on a chair at the back of the room. His hearing aid would beep, and his noisy breathing would sometimes become a sonorous snore, but he was there.

In the early morning, he could be seen walking the six blocks to a café, where he drank his daily coffee. On these occasions, he sported brightly colored pocket handkerchiefs—large, floppy squares cut from fabric remnants. One day I saw him in a local bookstore buying *The Tibetan Book of the Dead*. "I'm going to die soon," he explained.

A few months later, I received an invitation to his eightieth birthday party. It was a big party, and a hall was rented for the occasion. All of his friends and caregivers were there. There were congratulatory toasts, dancing, and a speech by Cyrus. The next day Cyrus checked himself into the hospital, where he died peacefully.

Toward the end of life, many people stop talking much. Maybe there isn't enough energy to speak, or the brain is processing very slowly. Caregivers often find it difficult to be with a person who doesn't talk. Most of us rely on words to fill up empty space, even when there is really nothing to say.

But quiet elders can teach us to rest in empty space instead of trying to fill it up. We can learn to go through our discomfort with silence, then relax into it. Words can be a way of distracting us from ourselves. With silence, we're confronted by our own wants and wounds. When someone is dying, a lifetime of buried wounds might arise—both the helper's and those of the dying person. You might not know whose confusion and hurt you are feeling, yours or the other's. We move on from it by providing what we can: the proper foods, personal care, a visit from a friend, sitting quietly. When Sharon was in a coma, I massaged her feet with lotion. My mind filled with images of my mother braiding my hair and washing my mouth out with soap because I'd said "damn." A painful longing arose in my chest.

For the family and helpers, the silence provides an opportunity to learn to trust themselves and to work on a more intuitive level. One daughter, who was always close to her mother, learned how to be close in a different way. She sat with her mother while they both read books. Every few sentences, they let their minds drift from their books to each other and to the space of the room. They made contact with the atmosphere as a way of connecting with each other. The room felt lively and full of warmth and awareness, without any words being spoken.

In the last few days before death, a person may not be able to communicate with the family or caretakers. She may be in a coma or focused on bodily concerns or simply residing in a world apart. If the dying person can't tell you what he wants you to do, you need to give care in the way that you think is best.

Lois was a dependable person. Her family had always counted on her for a loan or for advice. She'd had a painful life. After her husband left her for another woman, she became a nurse, and she began to overeat. But at eighty-three, Lois had lost her ability to be a helper. Small strokes had laid her low. She hallucinated that little people came into her apartment and gave her orders.

Her son, Tom, a powerful businessman, wanted to take his mother home with him so he could watch over her care and still go on with his own life. His mother wanted to stay where she was. "I would rather go to a nursing home than be a burden," Lois said. "You have to go with me," Tom said. "I'm too old to move," she insisted.

The next day Lois stood up from her chair, fell down, and broke her hip. The doctor recommended surgery. During the hip-replacement operation, Lois had another stroke and fell into a coma. The hospital put her on life-support machines. For weeks Lois lay on a bed in the hospital, with tubes in her nose and throat. The doctor didn't think she could recover. Twice Lois got pneumonia, and twice the doctors dripped lifesaving antibiotics into her body.

Tom wondered whether he should take her home and hire nurses around the clock. He had nursed at her breast; how could he turn off the machines that were feeding her? But he finally decided to do just that. Lois had told him repeatedly over the years that she did not want to be kept alive artificially. More recently she had told him she was ready to die.

Lois was transferred to a hospice respite unit in the hospital. As she declined, Tom cared for his mother. He brushed her hair and massaged the feet that had walked down so many halls in the service of others. He rubbed lotion on skin that had not been stroked for forty years. In her silence, as Lois lay in a coma, he was able to talk to her. "I resented your putting me in a boarding school when I was only seven," he told her. "Sometimes I blamed you for driving my father away." His voice sounded like that of a little boy. "Ma, Ma, can you hear me?" In those precious final days, mother and son passed over a divide of communication that is seldom crossed between two people. By the time of her death, Lois had relaxed and become a beautiful, radiant woman.

There are many ways for communication to take place. Leo was a very old man with a fatal liver condition. He was going downhill at home with his caregiver, John. Leo slept most of the day and prowled around at night. Then he reached a point at which he was sleeping for a couple of hours, then was up for a couple of hours, around the clock. One evening after his supper, Leo said to John, "You want me to die, don't you?" "Leo, I don't want you to go on like this," John answered. There was a clear moment of understanding between the two men. A couple of hours later, Leo fell into a coma and died the next day.

Sometimes caregivers don't want to let the dying person go. Mattie was eighty-eight when she began refusing food and water. She went to the hospital for tests, but the doctor could find nothing wrong. "She's ready to die," he said.

Mattie had only recently begun to bloom as a result of the circle of care that surrounded her. I wasn't ready for her to die. "It's not time," I answered. "Can't you put her on an IV?"

The doctor told me he had consulted with three other doctors, and they all concurred. When he had asked Mattie if she was ready to die, she looked at him with her gentle smile, squeezed his hand, then turned over and faced the wall. When he told me this, I realized that he was right. It was as if Mattie had touched the sweetness of life enough to realize that her journey was over. She had gone as far as possible in that body.

The doctor sent her home. Three days later, surrounded by her helping friends, Mattie died peacefully. Those who were with her at the end commented that she seemed to have more vitality as she was dying than she'd had before. "Mattie gave up her fear of life and her fear of death at the same time," one person said.

Working with Pain

Dealing with pain is one of the most difficult and heart-wrenching aspects of supporting the dying. Pain is never only physical: it profoundly affects the psyche as well—of the dying person and of the caregivers. Any physical or mental anguish that the elder feels can hardly fail to bring up corresponding pain in those caring for him. Your desire to do something and the helplessness you may feel in the face of the dilemmas involved can bring you to the point of desperation.

Helping someone in pain can be confusing. Some people feel a psychic pain and experience it in the body. Others feel a physical pain and experience it in the mind. Sometimes old people feel discomfort but are not sure where the pain is located. In the last few months of her life, Sharon kept saying over and over, "My elbow hurts." To her doctor, it seemed odd that her elbow would hurt, since she had stomach cancer. He tried different pain medications, but they didn't seem to help.

The caregivers thought that Sharon was remembering the pain of having fallen out of bed at the hospital two years ago and hurting her elbow. Finally, as Sharon became more relaxed in her care environment, her mind and body synchronized, and she forgot the pain in her elbow and felt the pain in her stomach. Then the doctor could treat it effectively; the pain medication began to work.

Dying people should have the comfort of medication that is appropriate to their circumstances. Ask the doctor to work with the medication until an effective dosage is found. Some types of pain are so severe that pain medication should be given on a regular basis, so the pain does not build up. Pain can be layered. When medication relieves one layer of pain, the patient relaxes enough so that another layer of pain arises. When a person is suffering from cancer or some other painful illness, morphine patches and morphine pumps can be used to release medication into the system continuously. In the final stage of dying, the mind disconnects from the body's pain centers, so medication may not be needed.

There are many different philosophies about pain and how to relieve it, and family members often disagree on the subject. I once took care of an old woman who had broken her hip. Her husband wouldn't let her take pain medication, because he was afraid she would act "goofy," and their friends might think she had Alzheimer's. Over the years, I have seen more families fight about how to give pain medication than about any other subject. Just the other day, I visited a woman who was dying. She was lying on her bed in her bedroom, completely relaxed and free of pain. In the kitchen her friend was arguing loudly with a hospice nurse about how to give the morphine. Her husband and other members of the family were slinking around the house wringing their hands.

One reason that caregivers might feel confused about pain management is that our society is in the middle of what I call the "pain wars." We have the technology to control physical pain, and also to sometimes reduce psychic suffering, with medication. What usually stands in the way of pain control is different belief systems on the part of those who control and administer the pain medication. Some believe that pain and suffering are part of the human condition—that pain, whether physical or psychic, wakes you up and teaches you lessons that you need to learn about yourself and others. Some people tend to overmedicate, reasoning that the person is dying anyway. If a caregiver has not worked with his own fear of pain and death, he might want to overmedicate the patient. On the other hand, some patients don't get enough pain medicine because the caregiver has a fear of addiction.

The elder's feelings, of course, are crucial and may differ widely. Some people have a low tolerance for physical pain and are terrified of it. They might want morphine when an aspirin would suffice. Others are afraid of addiction or of losing control. Some people want to be awake when they die. Others want to die in their sleep, no matter how that sleep might have to be induced.

Even health professionals disagree about pain medication. Some fear that their patients will become addicted, even though they're dying. Some fear that if they give too much too soon, the patient will build up a tolerance. At one time health professionals feared being sued for giving too much medication. Now there are instances of lawsuits for not giving enough. Someday there may be national policies and guidelines for all health professionals and training for all doctors and nurses in end-of-life care. But that is not the case now.

With so many beliefs, how can you as a caregiver know what to do? How can you give up your fear of administering what medication is needed and withholding what is not needed? Without clear guidelines, how can you let each individual situation inform you about how best to proceed?

Here are some aspects of working with pain and suggestions for embracing it within the circle of care:

See yourself as part of a team. Communication about pain and any fears about pain medication need to be aired and discussed in the team meeting. Try to come to an agreement within the care team, including health professionals and family of the dying, about how to proceed with the management of both physical and psychic pain. It helps to agree on one person who says what the dosage should be. Hopefully, this decision will be based on the expressed wishes of the dying person, but sometimes the person has not been able to express those desires. If this is the case, then the team must work together to make these decisions. If a strong family member is available, his or her wishes should be respected.

My advice is always to follow the doctor's orders—but you need to work with the doctor to come up with an effective policy and to meet changing contingencies as they arise. That requires giving the doctor accurate information, so he can prescribe properly. Many doctors prescribe medications "as needed," relying on the family to regulate the dosage. If you are working with a doctor who is fearful about medication, sometimes your own calm mind and good communication will be helpful. I've had the opportunity to work with well-trained doctors with enlightened attitudes, who have known how to medicate and how to cut back. Sometimes you can request a consultation from a pain management specialist, but such a person may be hard to find. The best method I have found is to work with hospice. A good hospice nurse will have the best chance of communicating with the doctor.

You might find yourself in a situation in which there is no meeting of minds. Then I think the important point is not to create a situation of pain on pain as a result of excessive fighting and struggle. Give in to the situation as it is. Calm your own mind and become one with whatever is going on. Then your calmness will spread and help soothe the pain.

Let the pain be your guide. When a person is in pain, sit with him and try to stay with his pain. Hold his hand or sit quietly by the bed. Don't think about anything else, just stay with the pain. Stay with the tenderness you feel for his suffering, then project your warmth and calmness toward him. If you begin to feel too much panic, purposely heighten the tension within yourself by tensing your whole body, then relax the tension, and calm yourself by giving the person some physical care. Notice the form of his body on the bed and the contrast of his hair against the sheets. The point is to let the pain open your heart and then bring comfort to the other and to yourself. Sometimes all you can do is acknowledge the pain and be willing to be there, in the openness of doing nothing.

Sometimes a dying person howls out with pain. It's important that people be allowed to go through that kind of loud good-bye. The howling seems to bring a kind of solace, the way a woman groans or screams as she gives birth to a baby.

When mind and body begin to separate, when a person has a foot in two different worlds, there arises an uncertainty that can escalate into fear. A loved one who is abandoning this life may get confused and feel that it is she who is being abandoned. She may feel wounded or angry. Often hurtful remarks are made to the ones the elder relies on most. Sometimes extreme agitation arises that is not a result of medication but of anxiety and fear of death. The person may become very restless. Depending on her physical condition, she may try to run away or, if bedridden, will toss and turn and move about. She may roll the bedcovers up and back, over and over. Often the pain people experience when they are dying reminds them of a lifetime of unresolved conflicts and suffering. Their minds may work with fearful speed. They may have hallucinations, not just of loved ones waiting on the other side but of frightening snakes or monsters. Sometimes they might feel they are being chased by enemies.

When a person exhibits extreme agitation, anger, or other marks of psychic pain, remember that the frightened elder is out of his body, confused and mixed up, and going through a real life experience.

The task is to help him settle down and try to find his "sea legs" in the process of dying. By using a combination of medication and communication, you can usually help the loved one through this frightening experience.

Watch for side effects. Painkillers can have side effects, some of which include nausea, diarrhea, constipation, and agitation. If any of these symptoms should appear, ask the hospice nurse or doctor to help manage them. There are medicines to counteract nausea and diarrhea. Constipation can often be relieved by a good bowel management program. Agitation can be caused by urinary tract infections, untreated pain, or metabolic responses to medication; sometimes changing, reducing, or rotating medication will bring relief.

Face your own pain. One obstacle to letting situations inform you correctly may be that you have not processed your own pain. Indeed, one of the benefits of working with dying people is that our own buried pain is brought up and out to the light of awareness. As caregivers, we need to work throughout life to get in touch with our own fear of pain, to learn how to be with that pain and how to see it in the context of our present lives.

We tend to block out painful experiences. To be effective helpers to the dying, we need to learn to lean into our painful spots, so that nothing is hidden from our consciousness. Situations can only inform us if we are clear about ourselves.

What has been your experience of pain? Contemplating this question brings to mind experiences of pain that I had buried. I remember the pain of a kidney stone. I had been high in the mountains for several days. When the pain hit, my friend drove me to the emergency room in the nearest town. I had been camping out for several days, was in extreme pain, and evidently didn't look too good. The doctor at the hospital thought I might be a drug addict and was afraid to give me any pain medication until I had been X-rayed. I waited three hours to get the medication. The pain scared me, and I felt helpless and frustrated. I was twenty-three at the time and had no philosophical basis for working with pain. Instead of trying to become one with it, I fought it and became tense and miserable. Finally, the doctor gave me a shot and apologized for having let me suffer. That ordeal was over.

Fifteen years later, after many years of training had given me a strong philosophical base, I experienced intense pain during natural childbirth. I told the doctor that I had changed my mind, I didn't want to have a natural childbirth. "Give me drugs," I ordered him. The nurse, an older woman who was retired from the army, got down in my face and said, "I've been watching you. You can do this! Your baby is early. He doesn't need drugs." Suddenly, I gave in and began working with my training and summoning my inner strength. I finally became one with the pain and pushed out my baby.

Other images come to mind when I contemplate pain. I remember the times when all my plans fell apart, when love ended. I remember how my mother looked right after she died.

Let such images arise. Lean into them. Let the feelings touch you for a moment and then come back to the task at hand. The contemplation of these experiences will help you as you work with the dying. It has helped me let go of too rigid a view of pain and how it should be managed. My first impulse is always to give medication. I remember the distress and tension of untreated pain, and then I recall the luxurious and liberating feeling of the pain medication taking hold. I feel that journey.

But if I am working with someone who does not want to take pain medication for whatever reason, I can respect that. If the person initially refuses pain medication but then changes her mind in the midst of pain, I can respect that. Or I can sit with a person in pain and not lose my own equilibrium. I know that people can go through pain and come out on the other side.

This is important contemplative work, and ideally it would be done by all of those who work with the dying. But not everyone has done this work, for many reasons—not the least of which is because, for some, this is their first experience of working with a dying person. That is why the team approach is so essential.

Pacify the environment. If the dying person is in pain and pain medication is not working, pay more attention to the general surroundings. Soothe the senses with lotion for the skin, moisture for parched lips, soft bedclothes and pillows. The best medicine is a calm state of mind. If possible, invite people in to meditate or pray in the room. Even one person with a calm and healing presence can set a tone of well-being.

LEARNING TO BE PRESENT WITH DEATH

Some days you'll want to be anywhere other than where you are, doing anything other than what you're doing. Working with the dying is working with feelings—the feelings of the one who is dying and the feelings of family and caregivers. It can be very trying. Caregivers often have a powerful desire for background noise, because the experience of being with a dying person—with all the emotions and fear and resistance it brings up—feels too raw. But opening to that experience is a road to freedom. We want it, yet we resist it. We throw up roadblocks. Anxiety and chaos are normal in the environment of the dying. You may feel some pain or emotion that has been habitually repressed, so you turn on the television, read a book, or create some distraction.

But avoiding being present is a disservice to both yourself and the elder. When someone is very frail and dying, he or she is usually very sensitive to the atmosphere. If the caregiver pulls back or spaces out or turns on the television, the dying person may feel rejected or left out. A precious opportunity has been missed.

Mindfulness of the tasks at hand and awareness of the environment will help you to be present and to establish the atmosphere of trust and stability that are so important for all concerned. Here is an exercise to help you develop mindful awareness.

Sit in a chair close to the person for whom you are caring. Make your posture as straight as possible, but don't draw attention to yourself. Notice the person lying on the bed and feel the texture of the environment. Is it happy or sad? Heavy or light? Then notice your breath. Feel the breath go out of your nose and into the space of the room. Then breathe in. As you breathe out again, your breath dissolves into the atmosphere.

After following your breath for a while, you might begin to space out and think of other things, like what you are going to cook for dinner or what someone said to you this morning. Whatever you are thinking, when you notice that you have gone away in your mind, come back and feel your presence sitting in the chair. In one flash, you feel yourself on the chair, you see the person on the bed, and you sense the environment. Then return to noticing your breath. If you do this practice for a few minutes at a time while you're with the elder, it will help you to stay more in touch with whatever is happening.

A more informal practice can be done while giving care. As you approach the dying person, breathe in his suffering along with your own tension at not knowing how to help him. Then breathe out peacefulness, as you very simply take care of the task at hand. It may sound alarming or even dangerous to take on another's pain in this way, but if you try it, you will see that all the pain of the situation will be transformed into a feeling of spacious ease.

When a dying person's world is chaotic, that chaos can serve as a reminder for you to calm down. If you encounter chaos, pay close attention to yourself and to doing the work before you. Be extra precise and deliberate. If you make this a practice, boredom and claustrophobia will give way to well-being. You will have found your inner strength, and that is healing for the elder as well as for everyone else.

If you become agitated when you are in the room with the dying person, tune in to the environment. Try using sensory awareness—what you see, touch, taste, smell, or hear—to take you beyond your struggle. If you are thirsty, check to see whether the elder is thirsty. Do you feel alone, isolated from the rest of the world? Close your eyes for a moment and listen to the sounds in the room and beyond. Pay attention to the details around you. Notice the way your tea pours from the spout of the teapot. Smell the aroma of lilies on the side table. Listen to the hiss of the oxygen tank; breathe in and out with the flow of oxygen.

If possible, try setting a definite amount of time to be with a dying person. If it's two hours, during that time put yourself into your work completely, whether you're sitting quietly or attending to tasks. Focus your attention on the person you are helping. Notice the atmosphere. Be aware of your own feelings. When your two hours are up, pay attention to your leave-taking. Don't forget to say good-bye. As you leave, notice any changes in yourself or in the environment. Do you feel emotional? How does your body feel? Then pay attention to your next activity. If you are resting, rest completely. If you are going to the grocery store, pay attention to the food and the shoppers and paying your bill.

If the situation demands that you go beyond the limits you've set for yourself, remain attuned to your state of mind and your body. If you are working at night and have to get up every hour to attend to someone, notice whether you feel tired. Do you feel grumpy or victimized? Do you feel exhilarated? Do you feel weak or powerful? Don't judge yourself; simply take note of your state of mind. This in itself can help you feel more calm even when no other immediate solution presents itself.

Tips to Comfort One Dying at Home

- Good bedside care is essential. You usually won't have licensed nurses around the clock, so you'll need to learn physical-care skills. Nurses from hospice, visiting nurses, and other Medicare agencies will generally train family and helpers in these skills. There are also good books on home nursing, some of which I've listed in the resource guide at the end of this book.
- If the person who is dying needs constant care at night, an overnight caretaker is a wise investment, so that the family can get some rest.
- Keep the atmosphere as relaxed as possible. Remember that relaxation comes from connection to the ordinary rhythm of life rather than from enforced quiet.
- Pay attention to the care of the dying person's mate, with good food and plenty of rest. Make sure the house is clean and tidy.
- Stay in close touch with the doctor by phone if she is unable to visit.
- Don't think you must reassure the dying person that everything will be OK. Honesty is the only way to establish trust.

Tips to Comfort One Dying in the Hospital

- Pay close attention to the care being given by hospital personnel. Most hospitals are not staffed to give a vulnerable dying person the level of care needed for maximum comfort.
- You may want to supplement hospital care with lotion for the skin, drops for the eyes, or whatever seems appropriate for extra comfort. When you give personal care, be sure to talk to the dying person about what you are doing, because the senses of touch and hearing remain active until the end.
- Advanced medical technology is part of the dying process for many people. Discuss with the elder her wishes regarding a living will, administration of fluids or antibiotics by IV, artificial feeding, breathing machines, and respirators. If possible, the one who is dying should indicate what approach to take, although when the time comes, it is often the family who must make the decision.
- Some hospitals and nursing homes have hospice or palliative care units, where patients can die with dignity and where there are support services for the family. Call hospice to see if the elder is eligible.
- Many hospitals will let a loved one stay in the same room; others will not let the family stay past a certain hour at night. Find out what kind of flexibility your hospital offers.
- Arrangements for what you want to do with the body of your loved one should be made in advance. If you want to sit with the body, request to do that ahead of time.

CARE STUDY

Henry's Last Gift

————◄o►————

Henry was a gracious and elegant man who lost his wife of sixty years to cancer. He was almost too gracious; he never complained. During his wife's illness, Henry slept at her side. When she died, it was as if he had felt her pain, struggled her struggle, and died her death. All that remained for him was the slow decline of his own body.

Henry's friends and caregivers tried to encourage him to live. They invited him to parties, tried to involve him in projects, and gave him love and appreciation. But Henry was not interested. It seemed as if his spirit had died along with his wife. Finally, he began to complain.

Grumpy, thin, and unshaven, Henry lay on his bed. He'd been to the doctor and had all the tests. "Henry is dying," the doctor said, "but I don't understand it. You have to die from something, and there's nothing wrong with him." Henry's helpers, knowing that he did not have long to live, called his children, who lived in other states.

Steve said, "Take care of him like he's your own father. I can't get away from work right now." Carol said, "I'm so glad I came to see him last summer, when he was still alive." They told the caregivers Henry wanted to be cremated. "We'll come in a month to pick up the ashes," they said, and gave the details for the obituary over the phone.

Henry lay on his bed breathing slowly. The doctor came to the house, looked at Henry's peaceful face, and seemed to forgive himself for failing to find a diagnosis. In Henry's warm room, the caregivers washed him, rubbed him with lotion, gave him sips of juice. Although Henry did not open his eyes, the caregivers knew that he felt their presence. As he breathed out, the helpers were bathed with feelings of love and appreciation. There was no struggle.

A month later, Carol and Steve sat in my office. "Those caregivers stole our father's watch," Carol said, as she hunched down in her chair. "We're missing a silver bracelet shaped like a snake," Steve said.

"You're missing your father," I ventured. Steve sat straighter in his chair. Carol looked me in the eye. "The caregivers have stolen your father's death," I told them as gently as I could. I knew they were in for a hard time dealing with their buried grief. They used hostility as a way to avoid their pain. They had to blame someone, so I took the blame. The police came, and I filled out the crime report for the missing watch and bracelet.

Carol and Steve had missed Henry's true generosity. He had given away himself, in the same way that he had given his possessions to his friends and neighbors. He had shared his moments of depression and grumpiness along with his kindness. The generosity of the dying is easy to refuse, but it can be the greatest gift of a person's life.

RESOURCE GUIDE

ORGANIZATIONS THAT PROVIDE
INFORMATION AND ASSISTANCE

Caring for the Elderly

Alzheimer's Association
919 North Michigan Avenue, Suite 1100
Chicago, IL 60611-1676
Phone: (800) 272-3900 or (312) 335-8700
Web site: www.alz.org

Alzheimer Society of Canada
20 Eglinton Avenue W., Suite 1200
Toronto, ON M4R 1K8
Canada
Phone: (416) 488-8772 or (800) 616-8816 (valid only in Canada)
Web site: www.alzheimer.ca
E-mail: info@alzheimer.ca

Catholic Charities
1731 King Street, Suite 200
Alexandria, VA 22314
Phone: (703) 549-1390
Web site: www.catholiccharitiesusa.org

Children of Aging Parents
1609 Woodbourne Road, Suite 302-A
Levittown, PA 19057
Phone: (800) 227-7294 or (215) 945-6900

National Association of Area Agencies on Aging
927 Fifteenth Street NW, Sixth Floor
Washington, DC 20005
Phone: (202) 296-8130
Web site: www.n4a.org

National Hospice and Palliative Care Organization
1700 Diagonal Road, Suite 300
Alexandria, VA 22314
Phone: (703) 243-5900
Web site: www.nho.org

End-of-Life Issues and Advance Medical Directives

I have found that the best way to prevent difficulties is to go over intentions and wishes repeatedly with the doctor, the caregivers, and all members of the family.

Let Me Decide
440 Orkney Road
R.R. 1
Troy, Ontario LOR 2B0
Canada
Phone: (905) 628-0354

Partnership for Caring
1035 Thirtieth Street NW
Washington, DC 20007-3823
Phone: (800) 989-9455
Web site: www.partnershipforcaring.org

BOOKS

Caring for the Elderly

There are so many more good books about caring for your aging parents than often appear in your local bookstore. Searching on the word *elderly* in any of the major on-line bookstores should give you more than six hundred titles from which to choose.

Silverstone, Barbara, and Helen Kandel Hyman. *You and Your Aging Parent: A Family Guide to Emotional, Physical, and Financial Problems.* 3d ed. New York: Pantheon, 1990.
A helpful all-round guide from a social work perspective that I have used.
Sparks, Muriel. *Memento Mori.* New York: New Directions, 2000.
A novel that depicts people in their seventies and eighties who go about their lives with the knowledge of their own mortality.

Creating Volunteer Care Programs for the Dying

Callwood, June. *Twelve Weeks in Spring: The Inspiring Story of Margaret and Her Team.* Toronto, Ontario: Lester and Orpen Dennys, 1986.
Capossela, Cappy, and Sheila Warnock. *Share the Care: How to Organize a Group to Care for Someone Who Is Seriously Ill.* New York: Simon and Schuster, 1995.

Home Nursing

Although the following books can be helpful, another method for learning the details of personal care is to call the visiting nurse or the licensed home health care agency in your community and ask to be trained by a nurse or physical therapist. The nurse will train the family or the caregivers in the best way to provide personal care in your particular situation. He or she will also train you in the use of wheelchairs and walkers and how to transfer a person from a bed to a wheelchair without hurting your back. Medicare will usually pay for this training.

McFarlane, Rodger, and Philip Bashe. *The Complete Bedside Companion: A No-Nonsense Guide to Caring for the Seriously Ill.* New York: Simon and Schuster, 1999.
Williams, Gene B., and Patie Kay. *The Caregiver's Manual: A Guide to Helping the Elderly and Infirm.* Secaucus, N.J.: Carol Publishing Group, 1995.

Dementia and Related Disorders

Alterra, Aaron. *The Caregiver: A Life with Alzheimer's.* South Royalton, Vt.:
Steerforth Press, 2000.
  *This beautifully written memoir gives genuine help for caregivers who are tak-
  ing care of their spouses. It conveys information on Alzheimer's, day care, home
  care, finances, and issues of relationship, and it portrays the state of mind of
  dementia.*
Bayley, John. *Elegy for Iris.* New York: Picador USA, 2000.
Grant, Linda. *Remind Me Who I Am Again.* New York: Granta Books, 2000.
  A memoir of a daughter whose mother suffered from dementia.
Mace, Nancy L., and Peter V. Rabins. *The 36-Hour Day: A Family Guide to
  Caring for Persons with Alzheimer Disease, Related Dementing Illnesses,
  and Memory Loss in Later Life.* Baltimore: Johns Hopkins University Press,
  1999.
Molloy, Dr. William, and Dr. Paul Caldwell. *Alzheimer's Disease: Everything
  You Need to Know.* New York: Firefly Books, 1998.

Choosing a Nursing Home

Many books on choosing a nursing home can be found on the Internet. Both
Amazon.com and Barnes and Noble's Web site (www.barnesandnoble.com)
have extensive listings of books on this topic.

Kidder, Tracy. *Old Friends.* Boston: Houghton Mifflin, 1994.
*Excellent book that captures what it is like to live in a nursing home. It conveys
  an essential sense of what it means to be alive*
Kranz, Marian R. *The Nursing Home Choice: How to Choose the Ideal Nursing
  Home.* Brookline Village, Mass.: Branden Publishing Co., 1998.

Death, Dying, and End-of-Life Issues

Albom, Mitch. *Tuesdays with Morrie: An Old Man, a Young Man, and Life's
  Greatest Lesson.* New York: Doubleday, 1997.
Callahan, Daniel. *Setting Limits: Medical Goals in an Aging Society, with "A
  Response to My Critics."* Washington, D.C.: Georgetown University Press,
  1995.

———. *The Troubled Dream of Life: In Search of a Peaceful Death.* Washington, D.C.: Georgetown University Press, 2000.

Leif, Judith. *Making Friends with Death.* Boston: Shambhala Publications, 2001.

Levine, Stephen. *Meetings at the Edge: Dialogues with the Grieving and the Dying, the Healing and the Healed.* New York: Anchor, 1989.

———. *Who Dies? An Investigation of Conscious Living and Conscious Dying.* New York: Anchor, 1989.

Nuland, Sherwin B. *How We Die: Reflections on Life's Final Chapter.* New York: Vintage Books, 1995.

Trungpa, Chögyam. "Acknowledging Death." In *The Heart of the Buddha.* Boston: Shambhala Publications, 1991.

Vermont Ethics Network (VEN). *Taking Steps: To Plan for Critical Health-Care Decisions.* Montpelier: Vermont Ethics Network, 1992.

This booklet, which costs $2.50, may be obtained by calling the Vermont Ethics Network at (800) 639-5861 or writing to VEN, Drawer 20, Montpelier, VT 05620-3601.

Webb, Marilyn. *The Good Death: The New American Search to Reshape the End of Life.* New York: Bantam Doubleday Dell, 1999.

A beautifully researched and written book that will teach you about the latest in pain management for dying patients as well as provide a comprehensive view of many of the obstacles that may be faced when dying.

Williams, Terry Tempest. *Refuge: An Unnatural History of Family and Place.* New York: Vintage Books, 1992.

Meditation and Contemplative Practice for Caregivers

Chödrön, Pema. *Start Where You Are: A Guide to Compassionate Living.* Boston: Shambhala Publications, 1994.

———. *When Things Fall Apart: Heart Advice for Difficult Times.* Boston: Shambhala Publications, 1997.

Cornell, Ann Weiser, Ph.D. *The Power of Focusing: A Practical Guide to Emotional Self-Healing.* New York: New Harbinger Publications, 1996.

Kabat-Zinn, Jon. *Full Catastrophe Living: Using the Wisdom of Your Body and Mind to Face Stress, Pain, and Illness.* New York: Delta, 1990.

Thondup, Tulku. *Boundless Healing: Meditation Exercises to Enlighten the Mind and Heal the Body.* Boston: Shambhala Publications, 2000.

Trungpa, Chögyam. *The Great Eastern Sun: The Wisdom of Shambhala.* Boston: Shambhala Publications, 2000.

———. *Shambhala: The Sacred Path of the Warrior.* Boston: Shambhala Publications, 1988.

Guardianship

Zimny, George H., and George T. Grossberg. *Guardianship of the Elderly: Psychiatric and Judicial Aspects.* New York: Springer Publishing Co., 1998.

Working with Gerontological Design

Bakker, Rosemary. *Elderdesign: Designing and Furnishing a Home for Your Later Years.* New York: Penguin USA, 1997.

Working with Color and Environment

Berliner, Helen. *Enlightened by Design: Using Contemplative Wisdom to Bring Peace, Wealth, Warmth, and Energy into Your Home.* Boston: Shambhala Publications, 1999.